COFFEE, TOBACCO AND ALCOHOL:

Theirs metabolic and hormonal disorders

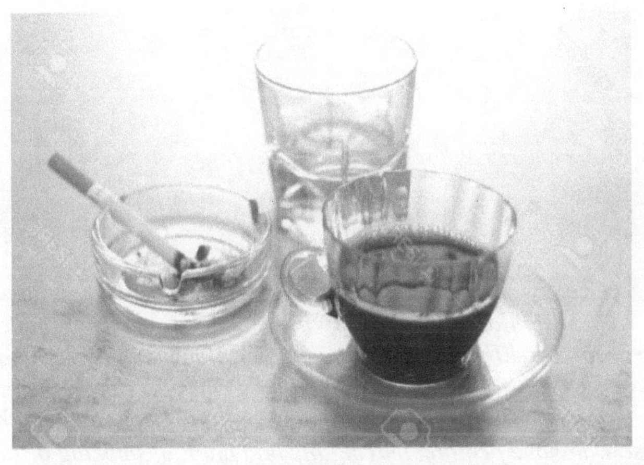

MARIO VEGA CARBÓ
Endocrinólogo

Primera Edición, 2020

To my grandparents: Ennodio, Aleida, Concepcion and Jesus
To my children, brothers, parents, uncles, nephews and cousins
To my wife Dr. Ethel Vado Osuna mother of my daughter Liuba Lucia
To those who enjoy a cup of coffee in the morning
To those who drink a beer or a glass of wine on a holiday
To those who have pending leaving the bad habit of smoking or alcohol

Table of Contents

Introduction

Coffee, tobacco and alcohol: *Theirs metabolic and hormonal disorders*

A drug is understood as any substance that has the capacity to act on the nervous system and create dependence for its repeated consumption. This very formal definition is normally associated with traffic substances and addicted people, however, there are drugs in your immediate environment and it is very likely that you get in touch with them on a daily basis.

Coffee, tobacco or cigarettes and alcohol are "soft" drugs accepted in our society, so we don't judge the fact that every morning we start the day with a cup of coffee or at a party we drink alcohol until we lose consciousness.

These "soft" drugs are not as addictive as a "hard" drug, which in addition to causing a strong dependence alters our body, but they could cause damage, perhaps not as quickly as it happens with hard drugs that are also prohibited, but Its long-term effect is worrisome given the high consumption in our daily lives.

Next, we will analyze in general the impact that alcohol, tobacco and coffee can have on health, then we will focus on the metabolic and hormonal effects that they trigger to finally outline the recommendations applied to their consumption.

It is time that we know how well or badly our consumption habits do to our health, which is our main treasure.

Dr. Mario Vega Carbó
Endocrinologist

Part I. Soft drugs and health

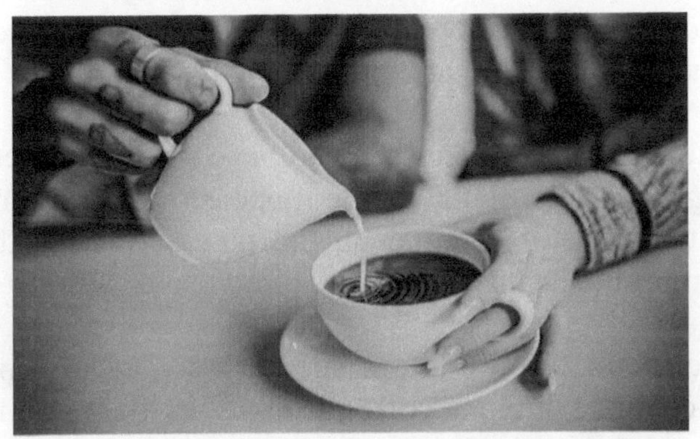

Chapter 1. Coffee and health

Coffee is one of the most consumed beverages worldwide, in fact, its annual production according to data from the International Coffee Organization, was 168.09 million bags of 60 kilograms for the year 2018 (1).

Such is the reputation of coffee, that we know very few people who do not drink it regularly, but its popularity is not an unequivocal indication that it is healthy, that is a very difficult assertion to maintain even when there are thousands of studies that try to reach only one truth.

On the one hand, coffee seems to have multiple benefits in each grain, which could be true if one considers the amount of antioxidants it has and on the other, it seems that in certain people its intake is counterproductive.

It is difficult for any health specialist to say to a patient "yes, continue drinking coffee as usual" or fight against the habit and do not drink a single drop" mainly because there are many cases and information about it.

Coffee acts in various ways in our body, for example, caffeine that is a psychoactive blocks adenosine which causes the increase of other substances such as dopamine or norepinephrine and manifests in the person more energy, a better mood, greater memory and shorter reaction time to stimuli.

Despite its name, caffeine is not only found in coffee, tea, cocoa and cola nuts also contain this substance to a greater or lesser extent and its effects are the same in any case. When caffeine is ingested, it is absorbed and passes quickly to the brain, does not accumulate in the bloodstream or is stored in any part of the body as it is expelled through urination many hours later.

One cup of coffee contains riboflavin, better known as vitamin B2, pantothenic acid, manganese, magnesium, potassium and niacin, as well as various antioxidants such as chlorogenic acid, caffeic acid, ferulic acid and cumaric acid, which fight the action of Free radicals

Caffeine does not represent a nutritional need despite its supposed benefits, however, if you think about the effects it has on the body we find the following:

Ingesting more than 400 mg of caffeine daily causes migraines and headache, in addition, this substance keeps us very active so we are prone to experience anxiety, irritability or nervousness, when ingested in the late afternoon or at night, it generates Insomnia and difficulty sleeping and resting.

The acids present in coffee can cause irritation in the stomach and intestines, in fact, it is recommended not to ingest it when a patient has suffered from gastritis, ulcers or has a sensitive stomach.

Coffee intake can also affect the kidneys, leading to the appearance of stones, affect the fixation of calcium in the body and increase the sensation of heat during menopause, also generates withdrawal symptoms when ingested frequently and suddenly suspended.

Coffee seems to have as many benefits as harmful effects, so it is difficult to decide whether it is a healthy drink or not. In this book we intend to analyze the most recent bibliography applied to specific cases, for example, the effect it can have on people with sexual, metabolic and hormonal disorders, in addition, if the drink itself can act as a promoter of pathologies of this type in healthy people.

Bibliography.

(1) International Coffee Organization (2018) ICO Yearbook 2017/18. Available at: http://www.ico.org/documents/cy2018-19/annual-review-2017-18-c.pdf

Chapter 2. Tobacco and health

Tobacco, unlike coffee, does not leave so much confusion as to whether or not it has any benefit to keep it as a habit because even the same cigarette producing companies warn about the harmful effects of prolonged consumption on health.

A unit of tobacco weighs approximately one gram and contains more than 7,000 chemicals, of which 250 are known to be harmful to health and of these 250, about 69 are carcinogenic.

Aromatic amines, formaldehyde, chromium, cadmium, benzene, beryllium and nickel are detonating substances for cancer and some are present in the environment, but all are found in every cigarette that is smoked.

That is why it is not surprising that smoking is the leading cause of premature death worldwide. In the United States alone, this habit and exposure to smoke generates 480,000 deaths, of which 39% are due to heart disease, 36% to cancer of various types and 24% to lung diseases, according to a report from the Department of Health and Services U.S. Humans UU made in 2014 (2).

In addition there is nicotine, a highly addictive chemical component and it is what produces that, despite being so harmful it is so difficult to quit smoking. You could compare nicotine dependence with the addiction produced by some hard drugs such as cocaine and heroin.

Naturally, a tobacco plant contains nicotine, but producing companies are responsible for making this concentration stronger so that it is sufficient to create and maintain addiction in consumers. In some countries, national legislation prevents the manufacture of these products.

When a person lights a cigarette and takes it to his mouth, nicotine reaches the bloodstream as it makes its way through the lining of the mouth and lungs, once here it travels to the brain in a matter of seconds. A greater amount of the substance is absorbed with frequent and deep mouths.

But as we saw, nicotine only fulfills its role to create dependence, the toxic effects come from the other 250 substances that come in that gram of product and the effects they have are really impressive.

Smoking damages almost the whole of our body, affects each organ and system, which decreases the general health of the person and increases the chances of suffering from cancer of the liver, pancreas, stomach, cervix, colon, esophagus, mouth, bladder and AML.

In addition, it also causes heart disease, strokes, better known as strokes, aortic aneurysms, chronic obstructive pulmonary disease (COPD), rheumatoid arthritis, osteoporosis, diabetes and exacerbates asthma symptoms.

In a woman of reproductive age smoking reduces the chances of a pregnancy, increases the risk of spontaneous abortion, ectopic pregnancy and premature delivery. In the baby the consequences could be low birth weight, cleft lip, sudden infant death syndrome and cleft palate.

Cigarette smoke is a kind of poison capable of staying in any part of our body and once there cause sometimes irreversible damage, even if we are not smokers. This is known as passive or second-hand smoking and is a combination between smoke from cigarette combustion and smoker exhalation.

The constant inhalation of this smoke produces approximately 7,300 deaths per year from lung cancer in the United States and just living with a smoker increases the possibility of contracting this disease by 20 to 30%.

The presence of tobacco smoke in the environment irritates the respiratory tract and has immediate harmful effects on the person's heart and blood vessels, increases the risk of heart disease by up to 25 to 30% and a stroke even in 20%

In general, mortality among smokers is almost three times higher than in people who have never smoked and their quality of life drastically decreases, that will be evidenced in the next pages that will reflect the hormonal effects of this common habit and harmful.

Bibliography.

(1) U.S. Department of Health and Human Services. UU (2014) The health consequences of smoking: 50 years of progress. Available at: https://www.hhs.gov/surgeongeneral/reports-and-publications/tobacco/index.html

Chapter 3. Alcohol and health

Alcohol, like coffee, is a very old drink. The Romans, the Egyptians and Greeks had their own methods to manufacture and store it, so it is not a new substance in our society, nor are the effects it has on the organism.

The exact dose with which a person can reach a state of drunkenness varies according to different factors, for example, age, sex, food, health status, exposure to medications, type of drink consumed and custom of the person, who drinks with More often you can spend more sober time, however, but this does not mean that you are healthier.

In general, excessive alcohol consumption in an adult man is considered to exceed fifteen (15) weekly drinks and in a woman it exceeds eight (8), with a drink such as 12 ounces or 355 milliliters of beer, 5 ounces or 148 milliliters of wine and 1 1/2 ounces or 44 milliliters of liquor.

Compared to coffee and cigarettes, alcohol is more problematic for those who consume it and even for those around them, since the judgment of a person is tarnished when they are under the influence of alcohol and are capable of taking actions than in other circumstances. He would hardly, for example, hit someone who barely spoke to him.

In general, the family nucleus is the most affected when one of the members has problems with alcoholism since it results in domestic violence, rapes, sexual assaults and accidents of all kinds, such as drowning, falls and even suicide.

Children who grow up in a home with alcoholic parents experience constant anxiety, stress, poor school performance and are more likely to have a problem marriage in adulthood, due to behavioral patterns seen in parents.

At the health level, alcoholic drinks also wreak havoc on the body from the first time it is ingested, but the strongest effects are evident over time, especially if the person has heart problems or hypertension.

Drinking alcohol frequently increases the chances of suffering inflammation and damage to the pancreas, an organ that secretes substances important for metabolism, also causes liver damage, which in some patients incurs complications and eventually death.

Similarly, alcohol increases the chances of suffering from cancer of the esophagus, liver, colon, neck and breasts and generates malnutrition because essential nutrients are replaced by the "empty calories" of alcoholic beverages, by hyperexcretion of vitamins, malabsorption of nutrients or effect of ethanol. In general, the B vitamins are the ones that suffer most from deficiencies.

A pregnant woman who consumes alcohol exposes the baby to suffer from fetal alcohol syndrome, which includes poor growth and poor muscle development before birth and vision problems, hyperactivity, nervousness and attention deficit in the child.

The brain of an alcoholic person is exposed to the loss of neurons and therefore, memory and reasoning ability. It also affects the nerves and the person experiences numbness and tingling in the extremities, erection problem and dripping when urinating.

According to a report published by the World Health Organization (WHO) in 2016, more than 3 million people died due to excessive alcohol consumption, which means that 1 in 20 deaths in that year were due to alcoholism (3).

This report indicates that three quarters of these deaths correspond to the masculine gender and that in general it could be considered as 5% of the morbidity worldwide, which is a regrettable fact if it is considered that there is no real need for alcohol.

With all this information we are ready to deepen the metabolic and hormonal disorders that produce coffee, tobacco and alcohol in our body, which after all the ultimate purpose of this book.

Bibliography.

(2) World Health Organization (2016) World Situation Report on Alcohol and Health 2016 Available in:
https://www.who.int/substance_abuse/publications/global_alcohol_report/msbgsru
profiles.pdf

Part II Metabolic disorders

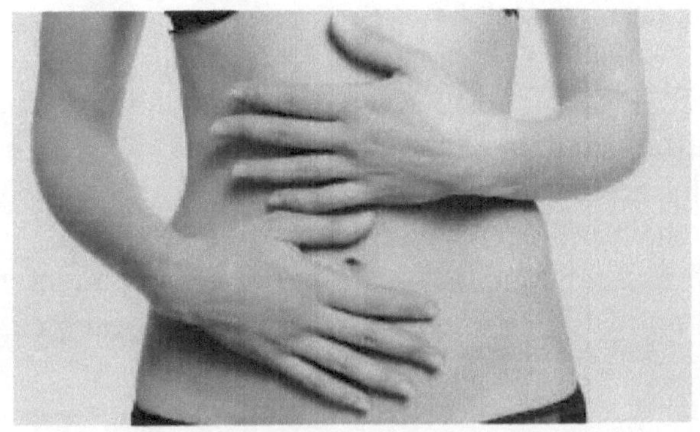

Chapter 4. Sarcopenia

The word "sarcopenia" comes from the greek *sarx*, which means *"meat"* and *penis* that means *"poverty or shortage"*, that is, shortage of meat and this is precisely what happens in the person affected by the disease, with the course of time loses your muscle tone.

Sarcopenia is a progressive and generalized disease that occurs in skeletal muscle and is characterized by a decrease in muscle strength and mass, in turn causing a decrease in physical performance.

This pathology is considered a geriatric syndrome and those who suffer from it experience weakness, loss of balance, difficulty performing simple movements such as getting up from a chair and decreasing the speed of walking. As it is a loss of muscle tone it is normal for the patient to also present unjustified weight loss and a sick appearance.

The quality of life of a person with sarcopenia is not the same as that of other elderly people whose loss of muscle mass is not as pronounced, for example, sick elderly people require more assistance, care and are more prone to accidents.

Since all the elderly experience a general loss of muscle to a greater or lesser extent, it is difficult to establish the prevalence of sarcopenia, so most researchers consider a muscle loss intense enough to produce symptoms.

Thus, in a study conducted in New Mexico (4) a group of scientists analyzed 833 randomly selected elderly people and it was found that female sex is usually more affected and that the disease increases the risk of disability from 3 to

4 Sometimes, regardless of the person's weight, race and socioeconomic status.

What causes sarcopenia?

Medicine and science have not been able to find the exact causes of sarcopenia, but several factors that significantly influence symptoms and are associated with aging are known, for example, inactivity and sedentary lifestyle, the reduction of the neurons they control movement and changes in the way the body manages the formation and atrophy of muscles.

Hormonal and genetic changes also play an important role in the onset of the disease, as do certain endocrine pathologies such as insulin resistance and chronic diseases associated with inflammatory processes.

Smoking and loss of muscle mass

Of the three products we saw at the beginning of the book, tobacco seems to have an important role in the development of sarcopenia, as evidenced by a study carried out by the University of Nottingham and the University of Copenhagen in Denmark (5).

The investigation involved sixteen elders, both men and women and at ages close to 60 years. To select them, their lifestyles were similar and everyone considered themselves healthy, with these parameters the group was divided into two, the first was comprised of non-smokers and the second by people who had smoked at least a pack of 20 cigarettes at day for at least 20 years.

The scientists intended to measure the synthesis of muscle proteins so each participant was given an intravenous infusion with an amino acid and one of the labeled basic protein components. They took muscle samples before and after the infusion and thus discovered that the rate of muscle protein synthesis, which contributes to the daily maintenance of muscle mass, was significantly lower in smokers than in non-smokers.

In another test conducted in the same study it was found that the amounts of myostatin, which is a muscle growth inhibitor and the MAFbx enzyme, which is responsible for muscle protein degradation, were higher in smokers than in non-smokers. This served to demonstrate that smokers have a much slower synthesis of muscle proteins, and therefore an accelerated muscle deterioration, thus promoting the appearance of sarcopenia upon reaching the age of older adults.

Bibliography.

(2) Baumgartner RN, Koehler KM, Gallagher D et al. Epidemiology of sarcopenia among the elderly in New Mexico. Am J Epidemiol 1998; 147: 755-763. Available at: https://www.ncbi.nlm.nih.gov/pubmed/9554417

(3) Michael Rennie (2007) More muscle for the argument to give up smoking. Available at: https://www.eurekalert.org/pub_releases/2007-07/uon-mmf070907.php

Chapter 5. Celiac disease

Celiac disease, also known as celiac disease or gluten-sensitive enteropathy, is a condition of the immune system where the main damage occurs in the small intestine. Affected people do not tolerate gluten and when ingested their immune system responds by attacking the intestinal mucosa.

Gluten is a protein that is present in wheat, oats, barley and rye, but it can also be found in commercial vitamins, supplements, hair and skin products, toothpaste and lip balms. A celiac patient should reduce contact with all these products and follow a strict diet to avoid symptoms, as it is a pathology that has no cure.

As the small intestine is the main one affected by celiac disease, the absorption of nutrients, vitamins and minerals contained in food is altered and the person may experience malnutrition, even if they eat in a healthy way.

What is the origin of celiac disease?

Research carried out in recent years suggests that celiac disease is a genetic problem, so it can arise at any age and have very varied symptoms, but it is not known exactly what triggers it.

Worldwide, approximately one third of the population has genes that predispose them to suffer from the disease and the odds increase by 10-20% in the close relatives of a celiac person.

In western countries about 1% of the population has celiac disease, while in Spain the prevalence ranges from 0.014% in the child population and 0.006% in the adult population, in other words, about 500,000 people could be affected but 70% of them completely ignore it.

Each patient manifests celiac disease differently, but in most symptoms it manifests in the digestive system through abdominal pain, and diarrhea. In other cases, especially when it comes to children, irritability and depression can be experienced.

In some patients the symptoms take time to appear or are confused with other pathologies, this happens for example, when the person suffers a deficit of folic acid, vitamin K or iron, osteoporosis, dermatitis and poor growth when it comes to children.

The intake of alcohol, coffee and celiac disease

A celiac patient is not prohibited from consuming all alcoholic beverages since it is assumed that not all of them contain gluten protein. Beer, which is produced from barley, is a product that the person should avoid at all costs.

For example: Wine is considered a safe alcoholic beverage for a celiac person, but depending on its processing it could be contaminated with traces of gluten and cause symptoms to appear. This happens with many foods and it is suspected that it also happens with coffee.

Coffee can affect a celiac in two different ways, the first is through contamination during grinding and the second is through a cross-reaction effect.

In an article published in the digital magazine *The healthy Home Economist* (6), it has been argued that proteins in other foods can sometimes cross-react with antibodies against gluten, just as happens in people with peanut allergy that they react to soy. It seems that coffee has this effect in some celiacs.

The processed coffee is the one that causes the most severe reaction of all and can trigger the symptoms even when the person is on a strict diet, this is because the protein present in the coffee is interpreted by the body as gluten.

This type of cross reaction is not the most common, but it is one of the strongest. It is also a high price to pay for a drink whose nutritional value does not appear as a necessity.

Bibliography.

(2) Sarah Pope MGA (2019) Coffee and Gluten Sensitivity: Never the Twain Shall Meet?Disponible en: https://www.thehealthyhomeeconomist.com/coffee-and-gluten-sensitivity-never-the-twain-shall-meet/

Chapter 6. Hypercholesterolemia

Hypercholesterolemia or high cholesterol is a condition in which blood cholesterol levels are above normal. The person has no symptoms, but the main consequence is the development of early arteriosclerosis and myocardial infarction.

Understanding hypercholesterolemia and the effect that alcohol and coffee have on it is a bit complex and requires a basic identification of the role of cholesterol within our body, we will deal with this in this chapter.

Cholesterol is a substance considered fat that is found naturally in our body, is part of the cell membrane and different hormones. Since fats are not soluble in water, they are transported in the blood by means of lipoproteins of different types.

Thus we find LDL cholesterol that travels in low density lipoproteins and if it is very high it tends to settle on the walls of the arteries forming plaques. Cholesterol-HDL is transported in high-density lipoproteins and is responsible for collecting cholesterol from peripheral tissues and arteries to transfer it to the liver for elimination by bile into feces.

After food intake the body transforms the calories that we have not used into triglycerides, which is another way to accumulate fat but now in the form of energy reserves that will be used in periods of prolonged fasting.

Cholesterol and triglycerides are not the only existing lipids, but they are those that are taken into account to perform a lipid profile or panel. When a person is said to have hypercholesterolemia, it is due to an increase in LDL-cholesterol or "bad" cholesterol.

What are the causes of hypercholesterolemia?

It is thought that hypercholesterolemia is due to genetic factors, since cholesterol is controlled by a huge number of genes that are transmitted from parents to children, but this family trend can worsen if a high-fat diet is performed, if you suffer from obesity or If you do little physical exercise.

There are some specific genetic diseases that are caused by certain mutations that produce very high cholesterol levels, such as familial hypercholesterolemia and familial combined hyperlipemia, but these are specific cases.

Coffee and cholesterol Does your preparation influence?

We know that coffee does not stand out for its nutritional qualities, in fact, it barely has calories and its content in proteins, fats and carbohydrates is practically nil but it contains two substances that increase blood cholesterol levels.

The cafestol and kahweol are lipids present in the oil derived from the coffee beans in a variable way according to the presentation and are transferred to the beverage in greater or lesser quantity depending on the method of preparation that is chosen.

Arabica coffee beans contain cafestol and kahweol in a larger proportion, while robusta beans contain half of cafestol and little kahweol in comparison and according to various studies, cafestol raises blood cholesterol more than kahweol (7) but the mechanisms of action that are generated are not fully known.

Both components are extracted by hot water, but they are retained in the paper filter by more than 50%, so they do not pass completely to the drink. This effect only occurs in paper filters, the fabric filters do not retain a large amount of these lipids and therefore would have a greater influence on the occurrence of hypercholesterolemia.

Alcohol and blood cholesterol

Alcoholic beverages do have calories but these cannot be considered a very influential factor in the increase of blood cholesterol, in fact, numerous studies consider that alcohol is beneficial to avoid arterial problems.

One of the explanations is that ethanol, present in any alcoholic beverage, increases the concentration of apolipoprotein A (apoA), which is a compound responsible for transporting "good" cholesterol or HDL cholesterol. This causes a decrease in the levels of LDL in the blood.

Many tests are still needed to prove this assumption and rule out other factors that could be responsible for this reaction. For now doctors and scientists remember that even the consumption of alcoholic beverages in moderate quantities has more risks than benefits, especially in people who have a family history and have already had high cholesterol levels at other times.

Bibliography.

(3) Gross G, Jaccaud E, Huggett AC. Analysis of the content of the diterpenescafestol and kahweol in coffee brews. Food ChemToxicol 1997; 35: 547-554.

Chapter 7. Hypertriglyceridemia

Hypertriglyceridemia is a condition characterized by excess triglycerides in the blood. Most patients do not experience symptoms, unless pancreatitis develops, but it is a side effect that does not occur in all cases.

High triglycerides are a widespread condition today due to poor eating habits and sedentary life imposed by the lifestyle of our society, where it takes a lot of time at work and preference is given to industrial foods rich in fat.

In the same person triglyceride levels vary with age, but a value less than 150 mg/dL is considered normal and healthy. When this figure is exceeded, the person is at a higher risk of suffering from coronary heart disease.

In a study involving thousands of patients (8), it was concluded that an increase of 1 mmol/l triglycerides increases the risk of cardiovascular disease by approximately 32% in men and 76% in women. If we were aware of this effect perhaps we would take more rigorous preventive measures
.
Why hypertriglyceridemia?

When some food is ingested and the caloric needs of the body are covered, the liver produces triglycerides, which can also become cholesterol when certain metabolic pathways are activated.

When you eat, the fat in food is digested and triglycerides are released into the bloodstream to be used during activities or to maintain vital functions. The part that is not used is stored as fat and the excess is reflected in the blood, but there are other ways to develop hypertriglyceridemia.

People who are overweight, for example, have more calories converted to cholesterol and triglycerides, which makes them more likely to develop the disease. As with people who consume oral contraceptives and certain steroids even if they maintain a healthy diet.

A liver or kidney disease, certain metabolic conditions such as hypothyroidism or diabetes, and genetics also greatly increase the likelihood of suffering from hypertriglyceridemia.

Of our three products to analyze in the book, coffee and alcohol influence the increase in triglycerides. Coffee, as we saw in the previous chapter, contains two substances capable of modifying a person's lipid profile, alcohol on the other hand, causes the liver to produce more triglycerides, which in turn limits the elimination of fat from the bloodstream.

Alcohol and high triglyceride levels

The intake of alcoholic beverages in large quantities directly affects the levels of "bad" cholesterol or LDL cholesterol due to how difficult it is for the body to metabolize alcohol, that is, the liver is not able to absorb it quickly and eliminate it.

The poor absorption and elimination of alcohol leads to an accumulation in the blood and these elevated levels can cause damage to the liver, as well as to the brain and heart. The metabolization rate varies according to the concentration of alcohol that the person already has, the health of his liver and the body's own capacity, which decreases as time passes.

Up to a certain dose, alcohol can increase HDL-cholesterol or "good" cholesterol, but beyond a moderate intake it increases LDL levels. This is because some alcoholic beverages contain phenolic and tannin compounds, which act as a cardioprotective.

Another effect of alcohol is that its excessive intake causes the body to absorb secondary nutrients causing cholesterol not to degrade or be eliminated and accumulate in arterial tissues impeding blood circulation to the heart and brain.

In conclusion, alcohol increases cholesterol and affects our health in an important way, so they should be consumed in moderation if we have optimal health and avoided at all costs if we are prone to disease.

Bibliography.

(4) Hokanson, John E, Austin, Melissa A (1996). Plasma triglyceride level is a risk factor for cardiovascular disease independent of high-density lipoprotein cholesterol level: a metaanalysis of population-based prospective studies. Journal of cardiovascular risk (SAGE Publications) 3 (2): 213-219.

Chapter 8. Adult Obesity

Overweight and obesity are disorders in which there is an abnormal or excessive accumulation of fat in the body. For adults, the World Health Organization (WHO) defines that a person is overweight when their body mass index (BMI) is equal to or greater than 25 and is obese when it exceeds 30%.

Obesity today is almost a pandemic. Only in the last forty years its prevalence has tripled and is responsible for cardiovascular diseases, diabetes, osteoarthritis and prostate, liver, gallbladder and endometrial cancer.

In 2014, a study was conducted in Spain (9) in which it was found that 39.3% of adults in this nation are overweight and 21.6% are obese. The prevalence of abdominal obesity was 43.3% in women and 23.3% in men.

The cause of this condition is very simple but it has great implications in our current lifestyle. A high caloric intake from processed fats and foods is more frequent worldwide, while physical activity has been significantly reduced due to working hours, transportation methods and urban construction.

As a result of this change in our habits an energy imbalance is generated between what we consume and what our body spends, and as we have seen previously the energy that is not used is stored in the tissue for prolonged fasting moments, but in our case They don't show up and those reservations remain with us and grow.

Alcohol and overweight

People who drink alcohol with some regularity can affirm that the contour of their waist increases during the seasons in which they abuse the drink, this is an effect known by all, what most ignore is that this long-term effect is a precursor of obesity

According to a European study on cancer and nutrition (10) alcohol consumption throughout life in men and women produces abdominal adiposity and a significant increase in waist circumference, but also in men it causes obesity with an increase in the rate of body mass.

To prove this, the researchers followed 258,177 individuals for nine years, aged between 25 and 70 years and covered ten European countries. In a second part of the investigation they tried to separate the influence between alcohol and beer by discovering the following.

Beer has more influence than wine for weight gain, but both have an important role on the appearance and accumulation of abdominal fat, specifically, men who consume more beer have a 75% risk of accumulating fat in the abdomen while that those who consume wine 25%. In women the risk for beer is almost double that for wine.

Tobacco, alcohol and obesity

In general, smokers are thin people and at the level of medicine, overweight was not associated with smoking, however, a recent study published by the International Center for Cancer Research indicates that the more kilos of overweight you have An older person is the chances of smoking.

For this study, genetic markers were used and evaluated about 450,000 people, discovering that the link between body mass index and exposure to tobacco may be due to common biological bases on addictive behaviors such as nicotine addiction and increased caloric intake.

This study was carried out as a way to prevent the worldwide incidence of cancer, but for us it serves as an incentive to review our behaviors associated with food and especially the products we treat in this book, which can lead to a difficult dependence on to break.

Bibliography.

(5) Javier Aranceta-Bartrina, Carmen Pérez-Rodrigo, Goiuri Alberdi-Aresti, Natalia Ramos-Carrera and Sonia Lázaro-Masedo (2014) Prevalence of general obesity and abdominal obesity in the Spanish adult population. Rev Esp Cardiol. 2016; 69 (6): 579–587

(6) MM Bergmann (2011) The association of lifetime alcohol use with measures of abdominal and general adiposity in a large-scale European cohort. European Journal of Clinical Nutrition, October 2011.

(7) Cancer Research UK (2019) Obese people outnumber smokers two to one. Science Daily Available in:
www.sciencedaily.com/releases/2019/07/19070221 1335.htm.

Chapter 9. Metabolic syndrome

Originally known as syndrome X, the metabolic syndrome is a set of disorders that occur at the same time and increase the risk of heart disease, stroke and type 2 diabetes.

Metabolic syndrome is not a disease, it is a condition in which the person manifests an increase in blood pressure, high blood sugar levels, excess body fat around the waist and abnormal cholesterol levels.

Having only one of these disorders does not mean that you have the syndrome and that eventually the rest of the symptoms will develop, at the diagnostic level it is considered that the person has metabolic syndrome when there are more than two of the problems mentioned at the same time.

Until a few years ago, high cholesterol and sugar levels were associated exclusively with adulthood, but the truth is that today children and adolescents present these problems in their body and are prone to develop the syndrome, in fact, 1 of every 10 has it and more than a third of obese teenagers.

What are the causes of this disorder?

Science considers that overweight, obesity and lack of physical activity are primarily responsible for the development of metabolic syndrome, as well as a condition called insulin resistance.

When a person suffers from insulin resistance, their body cannot take advantage of this hormone and therefore the sugar generated during digestion does not enter the cells to be used as fuel, then high blood sugar levels appear.

Genetic predisposition also plays an important role, those who have a genetic tendency to high cholesterol and high blood pressure are more likely to develop the disorder.

In children and adolescents the causes change depending on the natural processes of your body, it is believed that body fat and hypertension can be affected by growth hormone.

Tobacco, alcohol, coffee and metabolic syndrome

We are faced with a disorder that can be caused by the excessive consumption of tobacco, alcohol and coffee, as we will see when analyzing the next three investigations carried out under three different conditions.

In the digital magazine Circulation (12), a study carried out in the adolescent population of the United States was published, where it was shown that exposure to tobacco smoke increases the risk of minors developing the metabolic disorder whether they are direct smokers as liabilities

The researchers went to different medical centers and analyzed the blood of 2,273 subjects aged 12 to 19 years to get a nicotine-derived compound called cotinine, also assessed whether there were smokers in their environment and whether or not they themselves had the habit of smoking.

The results showed that of all the young people who developed the syndrome, 1.2% had not been exposed to tobacco smoke, 5.4% were passive smokers and 8.7% consumed tobacco.

For its part, alcohol is only missing two daily drinks to increase the risk of metabolic syndrome in an adult man, as evidenced by another study carried out in the United States (13) in which 1,529 people aged between 20 and 84 years.

According to the results of this research, those who drink excessively are at an increased risk of suffering metabolic syndrome, specifically, when men ingest two daily alcoholic beverages and women one. Those who consume alcohol in large quantities sporadically do not have a higher risk of developing the disorder.

And finally there is coffee, a university in Finland that studied patients with type 1 diabetes discovered that consuming three or more cups of filtered coffee per day represents an increase in the chances of having metabolic syndrome, that is, these people are more likely than the rest of the population due to their health condition (14).

This same research also found that those people with diabetes who would drink coffee in any quantity were more likely to develop hypertension, which for specialists meant a relationship between coffee and metabolic syndrome.

Bibliography.

(5) Michael Weitzman, Stephen Cook, Peggy Auinger, Todd A. Florin, Stephen Daniels, Michael Nguyen, and Jonathan P. Winickoff (2005) Tobacco Smoke Exposure Is Associated With the Metabolic Syndrome in Adolescents.RevistaCirculation. 2005; 112:862–869.
(6) Amy Z. Fan, Marcia Russell, Timothy Naimi, Yan Li, Youlian Liao, Ruth Jiles, Ali H. Mokdad (2008)

Patterns of Alcohol Consumption and the Metabolic Syndrome. The Journal of Clinical Endocrinology & Metabolism, Volume 93, Issue 10, 1 October 2008, Pages 3833–3838

(7) Stutz B, Ahola AJ, Harjutsalo V, Forsblom C, et al. Association between habitual coffee consumption and metabolic syndrome in type 1 diabetes. Nutr Metab Cardiovasc Dis. 1 Feb 2018. pii: S0939-4753 (18) 30046-2. doi: 10.1016 / j.numecd. 2018.01.011. PMID: 29501444.

Chapter 10. Non-alcoholic fatty liver

The non-alcoholic fatty liver is a condition in which there is an excessive accumulation of fat in the cells of this organ and is not due to an excessive consumption of alcoholic beverages.

Many patients do not experience symptoms at first but the progress of the pathology leads to severe problems such as non-alcoholic steatohepatitis, where widespread inflammation of the liver occurs and eventually scarring, irreversible damage, insufficiency and cancer.

Of all liver diseases, non-alcoholic grade liver is one of the most common conditions, in fact, 30% of the world population and between 70 and 90% of people with obesity or type 2 diabetes are affected. In the United States alone there are about 80 to 100 million patients.

Why does a person develop a fatty liver?

It has not been determined exactly why some people accumulate fat in the liver and others do not, nor are the causes of some fatty livers evolving until cirrhosis, but it is known that some conditions significantly influence the onset of disease by example, type 2 diabetes.

Overweight, insulin resistance, high cholesterol levels, high triglycerides, metabolic syndrome and high blood pressure are also health conditions that promote the accumulation of fat in a person's liver.

In some people, excess fat acts as a toxin in the liver cells, so there is inflammation of the organ and non-alcoholic liver steatosis, which is the advanced form of the condition.

Coffee can prevent disease progression

In other chapters we associate coffee with an increase in blood cholesterol, but when it comes to the accumulation of fat in the liver this drink can have a positive effect according to a study carried out at the University Federico II of Naples (15).

During the study, the authors used three different models with mice that were fed for twelve weeks with a control diet, a high-fat diet and a high-fat diet plus a coffee solution.

Towards the end they discovered that the daily dose of coffee resulted in an improvement in the biological markers of non-alcoholic liver steatosis compared to those who did not drink the beverage.

Coffee consumption in mice demonstrated a reduction in alanine aminotransferase, an enzyme whose levels rise in liver damage and a decrease in balonizing degeneration, that is, hepatocyte degeneration.

In addition, according to the authors' conclusions, coffee raises the levels of a protein called zonulin-1 'that decreases the permeability of the intestine and protects the liver from alterations.

Alcohol consumption is not advisable.

Currently, there is insufficient information available to advise patients with this disease about alcohol consumption, so withdrawal is recommended, since excessive drinking in people with metabolic syndrome is associated with an increase in progression of liver fibrosis, according to the Catalan Association of Liver Patients (16).

Tobacco accelerates damage in a few weeks

An article published in the journal Hepatology (17) showed that in obese rats with fatty liver the constant consumption of tobacco for four weeks worsens the disease by generating a mechanism called oxidative stress, where there is a very powerful inflammation.

The scientists wanted to discover the damage that prolonged exposure to tobacco can cause in patients with this condition and concluded that smoking in general produces systemic harmful effects that can aggravate any chronic disease and that it is most advisable to abandon the habit to have a better quality of life and avoid complications.

Bibliography.

(6) Vitaglione P, Mazzone G, Lembo V, D'Argenio G, Rossi A, Guido M, Savoia M, Salomone F, Mennella I, De Filippis F, Ercolini D, Caporaso N, Morisco F (2019) Coffee prevents fatty liver disease induced by a high-fatdietbymodulatingpathways of thegut-liver axis. J Nutr Sci. 2019 Apr 22; 8: e15. doi: 10.1017 / jns.2019.10. eCollection 2019

(7) Catalan Association of Liver Patients (2018) Alcohol consumption in patients with chronic liver disease and its treatment. Available at: https: //asscat-hepatitis.org/consumo-de-alcohol-en-P Patients- with chronic-liver-disease-and-your-treatment /

(8) Lorenzo Azzalini, José Altamirano, Ramón Bataller (2010) Cigarette Smoking Is Not Associated with Specific Histological Features or Severity of Nonalcoholic Fatty Liver Disease. Available in: https://aasldpubs.onlinelibrary.wiley.com/doi/abs/10.1002/hep.23749

Chapter 11. Gout and hyperuricemia

Gout is a form of arthritis that can affect anyone regardless of their age or sex. When talking about arthritis, there is reference to inflammation of the joints, which at the level of medicine can have several causes, but in the case of gout it is due to an accumulation of urate in that area.

A patient affected with gout experiences sudden and intense attacks of pain, swelling, redness and tenderness in the joints, especially in the metatarsal-phalangeal joint, which is located at the base of the big toe. The pain is usually more frequent at night than in the rest of the day, some patients show acute pain in the morning.

Being a form of arthritis, gout involves the degradation of cartilage that protects the joints and allows them to move smoothly. When this happens, the bones joined by the joint rub and damage, and cause pain, inflammation and stiffness.

What causes gout?

When a person suffers from gout, their body accumulates urate crystals in the joints due to high levels of uric acid in the blood, this is known as hyperuricemia. The body produces uric acid by breaking down purines, a substance that is part of the body and certain foods such as meat and shellfish.

Naturally, uric acid dissolves in the blood and passes through the kidneys into the urine for disposal, however, when the body produces a lot of acid or the kidneys excrete a low amount, it accumulates and results in urate crystals, which have a needle shape and surround the joint.

Joint pain and inflammation can occur even when the person has normal uric acid levels, this occurs in 50% of cases.

In general, gout is more common in men and usually appears between the ages of 30 and 50, while affected women show symptoms of the condition after menopause.

Coffee helps prevent gout

In a study carried out by the University of British Columbia of Canada and the Harvard Medical School (18), they tried to determine the effect coffee can have the appearance of gout in adults and for the relief of lovers of this drink, you can Help prevent its appearance.

The experts dedicated themselves to analyzing the data coming from an American health and nutrition survey carried out between 1988 and 1994, in addition, they carried out a survey of more than 45,869 men aged 40 to 75, who until that date did not present any symptoms.

Each participant answered questions related to their eating habits and alcohol consumption and by the end of the twelve years of analysis the scientists discovered that 757 men developed gout and that the risk was lower in those who would drink coffee regularly.

Of all the people analyzed, those who drank four to five cups of coffee had a 40% reduction in the chances of developing the disease and those who ingested large amounts of coffee reflected less uric acid levels.

Alcohol, a totally contraindicated drink

Avoiding alcohol intake is one of the most frequent recommendations that patients with gout receive, but it was still questioned whether wine could affect them given the beneficial properties in general attributed to the drink.

To resolve this concern, a group of specialists from the University of Boston, United States, examined the responses of 724 patients with gout who were followed up for nine years. 78% of the participants were men and had to answer questionnaires about their pain attacks, medications they used, diet, exercise and how often they consumed alcohol (19).

The results were published in The American Journal of Medicine and indicate that wine is one of the worst pain triggers in the male gender since the consumption of one or two glasses of wine increased the risk of suffering an attack in 138 %, and beer at 75%.

Patients with gout who smoke may have a heart attack

Smoking is another habit that patients are advised to give up so as not to worsen the symptoms of the disease, but according to a study published in Arthritis & Rheumatism (20) a myocardial infarction would also be prevented in this way.

Each patient with gout has a relatively small risk of having a heart attack associated with the disease itself but since it is an inflammatory arthritis, the increased risk may involve a substantial amount of myocardial infarctions.

This is due to the fact that the inflammatory phenomenon, together with smoking, increases the chances of cardiovascular damage, and of the 1,123 men who developed gouty arthritis in the study, 118 had an acute infarction and compared with healthy participants.

Bibliography.

(6) Choi HK, Willett W, Curhan G (2007) Coffee consumption and risk of incident gout in men: a prospective. Arthritis Rheum Magazine. 2007 Jun; 56 (6): 2049-55.

(7) Tuhina Neogi, Clara Chen, Jingbo Niu, Christine Chaisson, David J. Hunter, Yuqing Zhang (2014) Alcohol Quantity and Type on Risk of Recurrent Gout Attacks: An Internet-based Case-crossover Study. Magazine The American Journal of Medicine Volume 127, Issue 4, Pages 311–318

(8) Shuang-Chun Liu, Lei Xia, Jin Zhang, Xue-Hong Lu, Da-Kang Hu, Hai-Tao Zhang and Hai-Jun Li (2015) Gout and Risk of Myocardial Infarction: A Systematic Review and Meta-Analysis of Cohort Studies. Available in: https://www.ncbi.nlm.nih.gov/pmc/articles/PMC4521845/

Chapter 12. Hypertension

Hypertension is a continuous elevation of pressure in the arteries. It is a fairly frequent disease that affects approximately one third of the world's adult population.

In the body there is a pressure limit established as normal, this is because the heart must exert force on the arteries so that they lead the blood to the organs of the human body. The maximum pressure is given during the contraction of the heart and the minimum when it relaxes.

The increase in strength results in thickening of the arteries, which makes the passage of blood more difficult, this is known as atherosclerosis. The risk of suffering myocardial infarction, cerebral thrombosis or hemorrhage also appears, but can be avoided with proper medical control.

According to data analyzed by the Spanish Society of Hypertension, in Spain there are more than 14 million people affected and it is estimated that approximately 4 million of them have not yet been diagnosed. In the United States this figure is three times higher and the nation has about 75 million hypertensive people.

Why does hypertension develop?

The reasons why a person experiences hypertension are unknown, but several factors such as inheritance, age, sex, obesity, consumption of table salt, use of some medications and poor physical activity influence some people have the disease.

What happens to sustained alcohol intake?

Alcohol is a drink that can affect a person's pressure in several ways, even if the person is healthy and has not suffered any cardiovascular disease.

When more than three consecutive drinks are ingested, the body temporarily increases blood pressure as a natural response to alcohol and although these levels decrease with the passing of the hours repeated consumption can generate long-term increases.

On the other hand, those who consume a lot of alcohol frequently and reduce their consumption to moderate can lower their systolic blood pressure (the contraction of the heart) from 2 to 4 millimeters of mercury (mm Hg) and their diastolic pressure (the relaxation of the heart) of 1 to 2 mm Hg, however, stopping alcohol consumption abruptly does not have a beneficial effect.

When a person consumes large amounts of alcohol on a sustained basis, they should gradually reduce the amount they drink within two to three weeks, as doing so immediately increases the risk of developing severe high blood pressure for several days.

There is insufficient evidence to demonstrate a positive relationship between alcohol consumption and hypertension, nor is there sufficient information to determine whether the risk of suffering from the disease due to drinking is linear or increases with the volume of intake, so It is advisable to avoid it when the patient has been diagnosed with pre-hypertension.

Smoking and hypertension

The effect of tobacco on blood pressure does not give rise to so many variables and can be homogenized in the healthy population thanks to a study carried out in 2004 (21) in which it was shown that smoking significantly increases the pressure in a person healthy.

This effect is mainly due to carbon monoxide and nicotine present in cigarettes, which alter metabolism and increase cardiac work, coagulation and vasoconstriction. If it has this effect in healthy people it is clear that smoking is totally prohibited in people diagnosed.

Coffee, genes and high blood pressure

Coffee, thanks to caffeine, increases blood pressure levels in the body as occurs when alcohol is ingested, but the difference with this drink is that not all people can trigger hypertension and this is thanks to genes.

When the level of caffeine in the body is high the blood pressure rises and special enzymes come into action that will be responsible for metabolizing it and making the values return to their original values. Individuals who have the gene that synthesizes the CYP1A2 enzyme have the ability to metabolize caffeine quickly, but the same does not happen in those who have the CYP1A2 * 1F variant.

Thus, the latter can experience high pressure over time if their coffee consumption is excessive and frequent, as evidenced by the study in which it was found that people with CYP1A2 * 1F who drink three cups of coffee a day, They are 36% more likely to suffer a heart attack than those who only take one.

Bibliography

(6) Galán Morillo, Campos Moraes and Pérez Cendón
(2004) Effects of smoking on 24-hour blood pressure.
Cuban medicine magazine, 43: 5-6. 2004

(7) Hamer Marka, Williams Emily, Vuononvirta Raisab,
Gibson Leighc, Steptoe Andrew (2006) Association
between coffee consumption and markers of inflammation
and cardiovascular function during mental stress. Journal of
Hypertension: November 2006 - Volume 24 - Issue 11 - p
2191–2197

Chapter 13. Diabetes mellitus

Diabetes is a disease that occurs when the pancreas cannot produce enough insulin or when this hormone is manufactured at adequate levels but the recipient cells cannot use it.

It is a chronic pathology that affects the way in which the body uses sugar from food and unfortunately its incidence is high. In Spain alone, 11.58 new cases are diagnosed annually per thousand people and currently 13.8% of the population is already affected in this country.

There are different types of diabetes but usually two are considered as the main ones. Type I diabetes, more common in young people and children, is generated by the destruction of the insulin-producing cells that results in the cessation of hormone production, while type II is caused by a progressive resistance to Insulin is more common in adults over 40 years.

A woman can develop gestational diabetes during pregnancy, but the condition disappears after childbirth, as it happens in people medicated with corticosteroids, who by the action of the drug experience the disease in an induced way and once the substance is removed the effect It will no longer be present.

Why does diabetes develop?

Type I diabetes is caused by an autoimmune response, that is, when the immune system attacks the pancreas cells by ignoring them as part of the body. Medicine does not know the causes of this condition.

On the other hand, type II diabetes is closely linked to obesity because fatty tissue produces substances that decrease the sensitivity of insulin receptors, but genetics, lifestyle and physical activity have an important impact. Let's see how alcohol, tobacco and coffee influence the disease.

Women who drink alcohol are at greater risk

In Sweden, a group of researchers from the University of Umea (23) concluded an experiment that began in 1981 and aimed to determine how frequent alcohol consumption from adolescence to mid-adult age affected health, so participants They were analyzed from 16 to 40 years of age.

By 2017 it was discovered that women who maintained high alcohol consumption had high blood glucose levels and this is considered an important risk factor for developing type 2 diabetes, in fact, some women in the study developed the disease, but this effect was not observed in the male gender.

Researchers believe that ethanol is responsible for generating insulin resistance, which increases blood glucose, but what they have not been able to understand is why this effect is more pronounced in women than in men.

Smoking increases the chances of premature death

According to a study carried out for seven years at the University of Colorado, United States (24), smoking increases the chances of premature death in diabetic patients because it causes other health complications.

The study covered more than 53,000 Americans who were smokers or who are currently smokers and covered both healthy and diagnosed people with diabetes. It was found that the risk of premature death was double in diabetic smokers.

According to the results, women smokers with diabetes are more likely than men to die from lung cancer compared to women without the disease.

Coffee can prevent diabetes

There is currently a lot of controversy about whether coffee can really prevent diabetes or not, some studies suggest that a preventive measure cannot be considered while others, such as the one below, showed that it reduces the odds significantly.

Some researchers from Harvard University (25) analyzed data from a 20-year medical study, at this time, every 2 years, information was collected on the lifestyle, physical conditions, health and consumption habits of participants with The idea of evaluating the effect of coffee intake.

After 20 years, people who drank a cup and a half a day were 11% less likely to suffer from type II diabetes, while those who reduced their consumption increased the chances to 17%.

Experts point out that coffee contains phenolic compounds and that these improve glucose metabolism, so blood levels remain stable. They also explain that the drink contains magnesium, which is an element associated with the prevention of the disease.

Bibliography.

(6) Nygren K, Hammarström A, Rolandsson O (2017)
Binge drinking and total alcohol consumption from 16 to 43
years of age are associated with elevated fasting plasma
glucose in women: results from the northern Swedish cohort
study. BMC Public Health. 2017 Jun 8; 17 (1): 509. doi:
10.1186 / s12889-017-4437-y

(7) Kavita Garg, M.D., professor, radiology, University of
Colorado, Aurora; Patricia Folan, D.N.P., director, Center
for Tobacco Control, Northwell Health, Great Neck, N.Y .;
Joel Zonszein, M.D., director, Clinical Diabetes Center,
Montefiore Medical Center, New York City; Gerald
Bernstein, M.D., endocrinologist and coordinator, Friedman
Diabetes Program, Lenox Hill Hospital, New York City;
Nov. 22, 2016. Conference at the Radiological Society of
North America, Chicago.

(8) Harvard Health Publishing (2014) Coffee may help
reduce type 2 diabetes risk, say Harvard researchers.
Available in: https://www.health.harvard.edu/diseases-and-
conditions/coffee-may-help-reduce-type-2-diabetes-risk-
say-harvard-researchers

Part III. Hormonal disorders

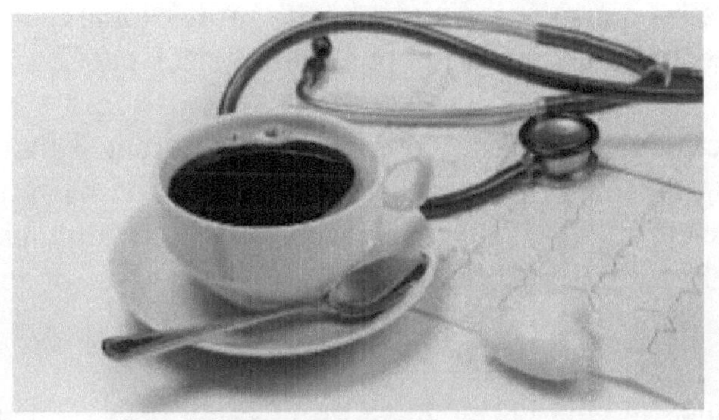

Chapter 14. Thyroid nodules

Thyroid nodules are solid lumps or aqueous buildups that form in the thyroid gland, located at the base of the neck, above the sternum. These formations are considered tumors because it is an abnormal growth in the cells, however the incidence of cancer is very low.

Thyroid nodules are not serious and do not cause symptoms in people, in fact, in 90% of cases they are benign tumors and the patient does not find out about the bulge until he arrives for consultation and a health professional makes him a respective imaging study or a routine neck check.

This condition is quite common, it is estimated that when turning 60 the vast majority of the population has a benign nodule of small size. In very few cases the nodules grow enough to be visible, obstruct the airways or prevent swallowing, that is, the passage of food.

In some patients the nodules produce an excess of thyroid hormone and hyperthyroidism is generated, but in general this type of bumps are benign whether they are solid or cysts filled with fluid and stored thyroid hormone.

Thyroid nodules that are benign and some patients do not merit treatment, just rigorous monitoring and medical surveillance to make sure there is no increase in size or other symptoms.

What causes thyroid nodules?

The medicine does not know the exact causes for which a nodule can occur in the thyroid gland, but it is known that there is a greater incidence in the female gender, especially between the ages of 20 and 40, which coincides with the reproductive age.

Hashimoto's thyroiditis, which is another type of disorder and the most common cause of hypothyroidism, is associated with an increased risk of developing nodules, but it is not considered the only responsible factor, it only increases the probability.

It is believed that iodine deficiency can also promote the appearance of these small tumors, but this lack in the daily diet is very rare because this element has been added in industrial products such as table salt.

Can tobacco, alcohol and coffee generate them?

To date there are not enough studies that show that coffee, alcohol or smoking are responsible for the development of thyroid nodules, but it is known that tobacco increases the risk of hyperthyroidism and that this in turn can cause tumors in the gland

Being a condition that does not represent a major health risk, most scientific studies have focused on other hormonal disorders related to this gland, as we will see in the following chapters.

Chapter 15. Thyroid Cancer

This hormonal disorder known as thyroid cancer occurs in the gland that bears this name and is located, as we learned in the previous chapter, at the base of the neck. Thyroid cancer originates when the cells undergo some genetic change or mutation and begin to grow out of control.

The disorder in a person's DNA allows cells to grow and multiply rapidly and not obey the normal cycle of birth and death, which leads to the formation of a tumor. In some people, cells invade nearby tissues and spread throughout the body. This applies to thyroid cancer, but occurs similarly in any variant of the disease.

There are different types of thyroid cancer, for example, papillary is formed from the follicular cells that are responsible for producing and storing thyroid hormone. There is also medullary thyroid cancer, which originates in the C cells that produce the hormone calcitonin. The most aggressive forms of the disease are anaplastic thyroid cancer and lymphoma, but fortunately they occur in less than 4% of cases.

What originates it?

It is not known what causes this pathology, but three risk factors are known. The female sex to be more prone to this type of cancer compared to the incidence that manifests itself in men.

Similarly, it is known that exposure to high levels of radiation, either by treatment or at the industrial level, increases the chances of developing thyroid cancer and certain inherited genetic syndromes such as multiple endocrine neoplasia or hereditary medullary thyroid cancer.

Is alcohol a risk factor?

Alcoholic beverages are not considered a specific risk factor for thyroid cancer, however, alcohol itself is a carcinogenic substance that can affect any part of the body according to the International Agency for Research on Cancer (IARC) (26).

This institute is responsible for classifying chemicals and agents according to their ability to produce cancer and classifies alcoholic beverages as "group 1", that is, there is a lot of evidence that they can cause some types of cancer in humans and they are not very far from the truth.

Excessive alcohol consumption is associated with cancer of the head and neck, esophagus, breast and liver thanks to various studies carried out in recent decades, but why is this drink dangerous? The answer is simple, thanks to the ethanol that is contained and the acetaldehyde that is produced in the body when ingested.

When alcohol reaches the liver, it decomposes and forms acetaldehydes, a substance capable of causing changes and mutations in the DNA of the consumer, which increases the risk of cancer of any kind.

Tobacco as a risk factor

Tobacco is not a specific cause of thyroid cancer, but it is cancer in general and is one of the most harmful products that can be consumed as it affects lungs, larynx, mouth, esophagus, throat, bladder, kidney, liver, stomach, pancreas, colon, rectum, and cervix, can also cause acute myeloid leukemia.

Whoever smokes or is a passive smoker has an increased risk of cancer because tobacco contains 69 chemical compounds that damage DNA and cause damage, cells grow out of control and cease to function properly.

Coffee can prevent cancer

For a time it was suspected that coffee could cause cancer because it was considered to contain acrylamide. Acrylamide is an organic compound that appears in vegetables when subjected to high temperatures, for example, when fried, it has been shown that this substance increases the risk of developing malignant tumors.

But an article published by the International Agency for Research on Cancer (27) showed that such a drink does not actually contain acrylamide so its consumption cannot be considered dangerous.

On the other hand, an investigation carried out in 10 European countries (28) focused on relating cancer consumption with coffee intake and rational differences, so the 520 thousand people studied were African-American, Hawaiian, Japanese-American, Latinos, whites and Native Americans.

Overall, the results showed that people who drank between two and four cups of coffee daily had an 18% lower risk of premature death compared to people who did not drink coffee and that they are also less likely to get cancer if they drink regularly coffee.

The researchers concluded that under the conditions of their study, mortality was inversely related to coffee consumption for heart disease, cancer, respiratory diseases, strokes, diabetes

Bibliography.

(6) IARC Working Group on the Evaluation of Carcinogenic Risks to Humans. Alcohol consumption and ethyl carbamate. IARC Monographs on the Evaluation of Carcinogenic Risks in Humans 2010; 96: 3-1383.

(7) International Agency for Research on Cancer (2013) The Acrylamide Working Group. Available at: http://epic.iarc.fr/research/acrylamide.php

(8) Gunter MJ, Murphy N, Cross AJ (2017) Coffee Drinking and Mortality in 10 European Countries: A Multinational Cohort Study. Ann Intern Med. 2017 Aug 15; 167 (4): 236-247. doi: 10.7326 / M16-2945. Epub 2017 Jul 11.

Chapter 16. Hypothyroidism

Hypothyroidism or underactive thyroid, is a disorder in which the thyroid gland does not produce enough of certain hormones involved in the metabolism, and therefore the body cannot function properly.

Because of this deficiency, obesity, infertility, joint pain and heart disease may occur in the patient with hypothyroidism, this is because the thyroid hormones control the speed with which calories are burned, the speed of heartbeat and activation of sex hormones, but people do not usually notice symptoms early in the disorder.

For reasons unknown to date, the female gender is ten times more likely to contract hypothyroidism than the male, in addition, it is present in 7% of women after childbirth and in 5% of pregnancies.

What causes hypothyroidism?

The most common cause of hypothyroidism is Hashimoto's disease, which is an autoimmune disorder where immune system cells attack the thyroid gland. Thyroid nodules, radiation treatment, certain medications, genetics and thyroiditis are also considered risk factors for the development of the disorder.

Some women develop hypothyroidism during or after pregnancy, this is called postpartum hypothyroidism, and it is because a lack of control in the immune system causes antibodies to attack the mother's thyroid gland, which puts the baby at risk of being born with problems physical and mental, such as autism, low birth weight or high chances of abortion.

Alcohol and hypothyroidism

There is not much evidence that alcohol is responsible for the development of hypothyroidism even though there is general talk of damage to the thyroid gland due to excessive drinking.

According to research conducted by a group of Ecuadorian researchers (29), the thyroid profile of alcoholic patients at the Center for Rehabilitation Center "Therapeutic Community of the Austro" shows that there is a certain relationship between alcoholism and the development of problems in the thyroid gland.

The study was conducted in a total of 40 patients, 30 of them alcoholics and 10 non-alcoholic people used as a control group, in general, the age of the participants was between 18 and 60 years. Each test was performed to determine the phase of the alcoholic disease and the values of thyroid stimulating hormone (TSH), free triiodothyronine (FT3) and free thyroxine (FT3) were measured.

With the results, the researchers concluded that of the 30 alcoholic patients in the study, 83% are euthyroid, that is, they have various acute non-thyroid diseases or abnormal thyroid function; 14% have subclinical hypothyroidism, which is an alteration in the function of the thyroid gland with very nonspecific symptoms and that 3% presented an autoimmune type alteration of the thyroid gland.

For these health experts it was undeniable the fact that there is a relationship between excessive alcohol consumption and damage to the thyroid gland, but they could not prove that a specific health problem originates, but that it facilitates other conditions in this organ.

Smoking affects the thyroid gland during pregnancy

It has not been demonstrated through direct studies that smokers are more likely to develop hypothyroidism, however, it was recently discovered that smoking during pregnancy affects the function of the gland in both the fetus and the mother.

The Journal of Clinical Endocrinology & Metabolism published a study (30) in which the influence of cigarettes was measured at two different stages of pregnancy: first and third trimesters. In both groups it was discovered that mothers experienced changes in thyroid hormone levels and that these were not beneficial for either.

When measuring the concentration of the hormone in the umbilical cord of newborns, scientists discovered that it was low, which is alarming if one considers that this hormone is involved in the baby's brain development and that its absence can lead to irreversible problems.

In another phase of the experiment the researchers asked the mothers to quit smoking to see if there was improvement and in doing so the hormone levels normalized and could be compared with that of non-smoking mothers. In this way they concluded that, fortunately, changes can be reversed quickly and it is possible to avoid complications after childbirth if cigarette smoking is completely eliminated.

(6) María Borja, Rita García and Diana Tapia (2012) Alteration of the thyroid profile in alcoholic patients of the rehabilitation center "austro therapeutic community". Available at: http://dspace.ucuenca.edu.ec/bitstream/123456789/2451/1/tq1002.pdf

(7) Beverley Shields, Anita Hill, Mary Bilous, Beatrice Knight, Andrew T. Hattersley, Rudy W. Bilous, Bijay Vaidya (2009) Cigarette Smoking during Pregnancy Is Associated with Alterations in Maternal and Fetal Thyroid Function. Magazine The Journal of Clinical Endocrinology & Metabolism, Volume 94, Issue 2, 1 February 2009, Pages 570–574, https://doi.org/10.1210/jc.2008-0380

Chapter 17. Chronic Hashimoto Thyroiditis

Also known as Hashimoto's disease, autoimmune thyroiditis or chronic lymphocytic thyroiditis, it is a condition in which the immune system has a defensive reaction against the thyroid gland and attacks it as if it were a pathogen.

The disease originates after an initial nonspecific aggression that sets in motion the proliferation of lymphocytes and the release of mediators, which interact with the follicular cells of the thyroid and end up causing their apoptosis, that is, their death.

The name of this endocrine condition comes from the Japanese doctor Hakaru Hashimoto, who made the first description in 1912 and called it a lymphomatous goiter. The term "thyroiditis" is also used but this is because the attack of the immune system causes inflammation of the gland and that it acquires a more voluminous size.

As the thyroid is part of the endocrine system, it produces and coordinates many important bodily functions, so its failure causes various problems in the body, including other diseases such as hypothyroidism. In some cases, Hashimoto's disease presents with adrenal insufficiency and type 1 diabetes and is part of a condition called autoimmune polyglandular syndrome type 2 (PGAII).

Middle-aged women are more prone to autoimmune thyroiditis, but it is also possible that it appears in men, children, young people and the elderly. In any case, the symptoms take from months to years to perceive and over time the capacity of the thyroid gland is greatly reduced.

What causes Hashimoto's disease?

To date it is not known what exactly causes the immune response that triggers Hashimoto's disease. Some scientists believe that a virus or a bacterium could be responsible for this reaction in the body, others relate the symptoms to a genetic failure, as is the case with other immune diseases such as rheumatoid arthritis.

For now it is considered that both hereditary factors, such as sex and age of the person determine the probability of the disorder, therefore, it is more common for an affected patient to have relatives in similar conditions.

Coffee and alcohol are not listed as triggers of this disease, there are no indications that they improve or help prevent it, however, smoking does have some influence and we will see that below.

Smoking and Hashimoto's disease

Smoking affects the function of the thyroid gland in a generalized way and can create multiple abnormalities according to a study published more than twenty years ago in The New England Journal of Medicine (31).

The researchers in charge concentrated on studying women smokers with hypothyroidism and discovered that the habit, thanks to the amount of toxic substances transmitted to the body, further decreases the secretion of the hormone and its effect on the body. In women with subclinical hypothyroidism, the cigarette exacerbated the hormone deficiency and this was evidenced in lower serum concentrations.

Smoking patients with Hashimoto's disease are also more likely to have a failure in the gland and hence the development of hypothyroidism, but this is specifically due to the cyanide present in tobacco smoke.

Cyanide is released from cigarettes the moment they are lit and once inside the body it becomes thiocyanate, which acts as an antithyroid agent and inhibits iodine uptake and thyroid hormone synthesis.

So tobacco is not directly responsible for Hashimoto's disease, but it can facilitate the conditions for a more pronounced hormone failure, that is, hypothyroidism, which in most cases derives from this disease.

Bibliography.

(8) Robert D. Utiger, M.D (1995) Cigarette Smoking and the Thyroid. Revista The New England Journal of Medicine 1995; 333:1001-1002 DOI: 10.1056/NEJM199510123331510

Chapter 18. Hyperthyroidism

Hyperthyroidism, also known as overactive thyroid, is a disorder in which the thyroid gland produces an excess of hormones and as a consequence in the body there are widespread changes in vital systems.

The thyroid function is to produce several hormones, including thyroxine (T4) and triiodothyronine (T3), which are responsible for controlling the use of fats and carbohydrates, body temperature, heart rate and protein production.

When a person suffers from hyperthyroidism all these functions are accelerated due to the excess of the thyroxine hormone, so he experiences a sudden weight loss, sweating, palpitations, difficulty sleeping, changes in the thickness and amount of hair, muscle weakness and a irritable mood

This condition manifests itself in approximately 1% of the world population, and occurs mainly in women between 30 and 40 years of age, patients with other thyroid problems and people over 60 years.

As it is a disease that affects the body's vital systems, its evolution involves other problems such as congestive heart failure and osteoporosis, but the symptoms are not noticeable at first.

Why does a person suffer from hyperthyroidism?

A person can develop hypothyroidism because of a thyroid-related disease, for example, Plummer's disease, where the gland is atrophied by the excess production of thyroid hormone and the appearance of a multinodular goiter.

Graves' disease, which is an autoimmune disorder, produces too many T4-stimulating antibodies, which also induces hyperthyroidism. It is common for this disorder to affect several members of the same family, so it is considered that there is a genetic cause.

When thyroid inflammation occurs after pregnancy, the mother is likely to develop the disease because of an autoimmune response or for unknown reasons. The inflammation prevents the storage of the F4 and this being unable to occupy the place moves to the bloodstream.

So far there are no studies that show that coffee consumption increases the chances of developing hyperthyroidism, nor protects the body and can affect it if the person is already sick.

With tobacco, studies have not been conclusive, but it has been shown that excessive drinking affects the thyroid gland in a certain way.

A person with hyperthyroidism should avoid alcohol

A study published in the magazine 'The Lancet' (32) showed that the daily amount of alcohol established as healthy can actually be harmful when mixed with other factors, for example, social habits around drinking.

The researchers carried out a meta-analysis of 83 studies carried out in 19 industrialized countries and in total they had 600,000 regular consumers of liquor. The data gathered from the participants were their age, sex, tobacco consumption, incidence of diabetes, cardiovascular diseases and amount of alcohol ingested in one year.

According to their findings, more than 100 grams of pure alcohol per week shortens life expectancy significantly and each drink taken over this limit subtracts 30 minutes of life, increases the risk of strokes, aneurysms and heart failure.

According to the scientists, each more cup that is taken from that limit shortens life by 30 minutes; In addition to increasing the risk of strokes, severe aneurysms and heart failure, among others. And in that sense, the researchers' conclusion is that countries adopt lower limits of recommended alcohol consumption.

This information was contrasted with the recommendations in the countries involved in the study and it was discovered that in countries such as Spain, Portugal and Italy, where a daily limit was established based on their customs, it exceeds almost four times the amount that is actually healthy.

The experts concluded that since the recommended values are intended for absolutely healthy people, people with liver disorders, cirrhosis, acute inflammatory processes, diabetes, hyperthyroidism, and kidney problems should completely refrain from drinking, as they showed that there is no an amount that can be considered healthy.

Bibliography.

(9) Angela M Wood, Stephen Kaptoge, Adam S Butterworth, Peter Willeit, Samantha Warnakula, Thomas Bolton (2018) Risk thresholds for alcohol consumption: combined analysis of individual-participant data for 599 912 current drinkers in 83 prospective studies. Magazine The Lancet Volume 391, ISSUE 10129, P1513-1523, APRIL 14, 2018

Chapter 19. Osteoporosis

Osteoporosis is a disease in which the generation of bones is slower and therefore there is a decrease in bone mass density, making the skeleton of the person much more fragile and susceptible to fractures.

Bone is not an inert entity, as you might think thanks to its hardness, it is actually living tissue that is constantly decomposing and replacing, so every seven or ten years we have bones completely regenerated by our body.

When a person suffers from osteoporosis, his body does not restore the bones with the same efficiency so that they become more porous, the number and size of the internal cavities increases and they break more easily.

Anyone can suffer from this disease, but there is a higher incidence in white and Asian women who are over 60 years of age due to hormonal changes experienced by the female body during menopause.

Why does a person get sick with osteoporosis?

Bone formation and maintenance is mediated by destructive and constructive phases, which in turn are determined by hormones, when hormonal activity is impaired begins poor bone formation and marks the onset of osteoporosis.

Diet, unhealthy habits, the amount of vitamin D and exercise are factors that cause the loss or gain of bone density, for example, regular physical activity, which could be considered a risk for weak bones, serves as a stimulus for Calcium fixation and strengthens the bone structure in general, not just the part that is exercised.

A healthy person reaches the maximum possible bone density near 30-35 years, from that moment, naturally a loss of bone mass is not triggered, not serious or dangerous for the individual. In women the bone density that is reached is lower and during menopause bone loss is accelerated, so this disease appears more in women.

Bones and coffee consumption

Excessive coffee consumption could increase the risk of osteoporosis because it can accelerate bone loss due to caffeine. This substance has the ability to make osteoblasts, the cells involved in bone formation, less efficient and can even kill them. It also affects the absorption of calcium in the intestine, according to an article published in the Journal of Orthopedic Surgery and Research (33).

This effect is not unique to coffee, any beverage with caffeine does the same, so the consumption of tea, soft drinks and infusions of yerba mate are not healthier since they also contain caffeine and as added xanthines, which promote the excretion of calcium by the urine.

Alcohol and osteoporosis

Alcohol consumption is also not favorable when we talk about bone health, even in young people. According to a Course of Osteoporosis and Bone Metabolic Pathology dictated by the Spanish Society of Rheumatology (SER) (34), young men who overdo drinking weaken their skeletal system and become more prone to suffer from this disease.

The experts of this institution explain that in men there are three possible causes for osteoporosis, the first is the consumption of alcohol, which has toxic effects on the bones and affects their formation and quality.

Secondly there are corticosteroid treatments and ultimately hypogonadism, which is the failure of the male hormone due to some disease.

Osteoporosis and smoking

It has long been known that tobacco is an important risk factor for the development of osteoporosis mainly because it affects the metabolism of calcium and vitamin D, induces estrogen reduction and increases the amount of androgens (35).

In general, adults over 60 who still smoke are 30% to 40% more likely to have a broken hip than non-smokers of the same age, but bone wear due to tobacco can begin at any age.

The ways in which cigarettes affect bones are many, for example:

• Reduces the supply of oxygen to the bones and other tissues of the body.
• Decomposes estrogen in the body more quickly and this hormone is involved in bone building and maintenance, both in men and women.
• Prevents wound healing and fracture consolidation.
• It is associated with an increased risk of low back pain and rheumatoid arthritis.
• Causes excessive thinness and weakness.

It seems that the health of our bones is more delicate than we think. Our three products studied in the book promote the appearance of osteoporosis to a greater or lesser extent, with alcohol and tobacco being totally contraindicated and coffee should be taken in moderate daily amounts.

Bibliography.

(9) Julia Thomson (2006) What that daily COFFE is really doing to your BODY. Disponibleen: https://www.pressreader.com/uk/daily-mail/20150310/282329678409435

(10) Infosalud (2019) La ingesta elevada de alcohol, una de las principales causas de osteoporosis entre los hombres, según expertos. Disponible en: https://www.infosalus.com/salud-investigacion/noticia-ingesta-elevada-alcohol-principales-causas-osteoporosis-hombres-expertos-20190218120158.html

(11) Judith S. Brand, Mei-Fen Chan, Mitch Dowsett, Elizabeth Folkerd, Nicholas J. Wareham, Robert N. Luben, Yvonne T. van der Schouw, Kay-TeeKhaw (2011) Cigarette Smoking and Endogenous Sex Hormones in PostmenopausalWomen. The Journal of Clinical Endocrinology & Metabolism, Volume 96, Issue 10, 1 October 2011, Pages 3184–3192

Chapter 20 Lipotimias

Lipotimia is a temporary fainting due to a decrease in blood flow to the brain. The recovery after this sensation is spontaneous and happens completely, that is, the person returns to normal and does not feel any other symptoms or discomfort.

Lipotimia and syncope are usually confused, but each refers to a different situation. When someone has a lipotimia they experience a feeling of fainting, there are previous symptoms and there is no loss of consciousness. On the other hand, a syncope does not show symptoms but occurs unexpectedly and there is a loss of consciousness or fainting.

Before a lipotimia there is cold sweating, generalized weakness, visual disturbances, nausea, lightheadedness and a sensation of heat on the face, all these symptoms become more acute and then disappear in a matter of a couple of minutes.

Why do lipotimia occur?

Neither lipotimia nor syncope are a disease or disorder, they are transient reactions that can occur due to anxiety, fever, excess heat, stress, strong emotions or blood draws. In some people a simple injection triggers a lipotimia, but the effect passes as soon as the procedure ends.

Syncope can be caused by very strong emotions, blows, lack of oxygen and poor food, for example, it is common for a person who does not eat breakfast faints due to lack of glucose, which is the energy used by the brain.

Likewise, a syncope can be the product of cardiac problems, such as ventricular and supraventricular tachycardia, sinus node dysfunction and hypertrophic cardiomyopathy.

There is no evidence that tobacco can generate syncope or lipotimia, it only creates the sensation of dizziness when people smoke for the first time or smoke a cigarette after having quit for a long time. Coffee and especially alcohol can cause someone to fade if ingested in large quantities.

Coffee can affect blood flow to the brain

The caffeine in coffee raises the heart rate when ingested in moderate doses, but this increase does not pose a threat to cardiovascular health as long as the consumption is not exceeded above the daily 5 cups.

In fact, drinking about 3 cups of the drink per day allows you to keep your heartbeat at an adequate rate, but according to research published in Human Brain Mapping (33) drinking more than 960 milligrams of coffee per day would affect circulation, making heavier blood in the long term and making the person feel dizzy and eventually experience lipotimia.

Alcohol induces fainting and loss of consciousness

The vast majority of people know that after excessive alcohol intake some drinkers faint spontaneously, but they completely ignore the biological mechanisms behind this reaction.
When the level of alcohol in the blood is excessively high the person may faint or fade momentarily but in both cases a memory failure is created and the person is unable to remember what he did a few hours after overcoming the state of drunkenness.

According to a study carried out by the Alcoholism Research Society (34), in the brain there is a region called the hippocampus, which is very sensitive to alcohol and is responsible for the formation of new memories. Excess blood alcohol limits the capacity of the hippocampus, so no memories are created and because of this the person thinks they don't remember anything the next day during the hangover, but memories never really formed.

Researchers at the Alcoholism Research Society explain that during a loss of consciousness, physical damage can be caused by a fall that leads to fractures, but these brain "blackouts" can also cause significant psychological damage when linked to neurobiological abnormalities and psychiatric symptoms. .

The response to alcohol is different in each person and only lipotimia or syncope can occur after the abuse of the drink, which as we have seen throughout the book is not recommended in any way.

Bibliography.

(12) Rachel Moss (2017) Why do we blackout when drunk? everything you need to know about alcohol-related memory loss. Disponibleen: https://www.huffingtonpost.co.uk

(13) Reagan R, Kim Fromme (2016)Alcohol-induced blackouts: A review of recent clinical research with practical implications and recommendations for future studies. Alcohol ClinExp Res. PMC 2017 May 1

Chapter 21. Adrenal insufficiency

Adrenal insufficiency is a condition that occurs when the adrenal glands produce fewer hormones than they should. In this disorder the person does not experience symptoms or discomfort until he reaches a point of crisis where he perceives tiredness, abdominal pain, sweating, nausea and changes in the skin.

Renal insufficiency is not the same as adrenal insufficiency, the latter refers to the failure of the renal glands that are just above the kidneys and are responsible for producing hormones that control blood pressure and balance the levels of mineral salts in the body.

According to The Journal of Clinical Endocrinology & Metabolism (38), it is uncommon for a person to suffer from a failure in the renal glands, in fact, the annual incidence is 4-6 new patients for every one hundred thousand people and only one doctor Endocrinologist can diagnose it by standard test procedures.

What is Addison's disease?

There are two types of adrenal insufficiency and Addison's disease is one of them. In this case, the renal glands do not produce enough cortisol and aldosterone due to autoimmune damage or a genetic problem, this is also known as primary adrenal insufficiency.

In central adrenal insufficiency, the problem lies in the pituitary gland of the brain, which does not produce enough adrenocorticotropin (ACTH), which is a hormone that activates the production of cortisol in the adrenal glands.

Some people may have temporary adrenal insufficiency if they ingest high doses of cortisol-like medications, such as prednisone used in rheumatic processes. Here the effect on the glands occurs when the administration of the drug is interrupted or suddenly reduced.

What causes adrenal insufficiency?

Addison's disease occurs when the body's defense system attacks and destroys the tissues of the adrenal glands, thanks to the damage they cannot produce hormones. It is also possible that it is caused by an injury in this area, by an infection and by certain genetic diseases.

In the case of central adrenal insufficiency, the failure may be due to the consumption of drugs similar to predisone, for example, hydrocortisone and dexamethasone, it may also be due to birth problems, infections, tumors or injuries caused by surgery and radiation.

Currently there are no studies that show that coffee, alcohol and smoking can cause adrenal insufficiency in a person, nor has it been scientifically proven that they are able to prevent, improve or worsen symptoms.

Bibliography.

(14) Baha Arafah, Richard Auchus (2010) Adrenal insufficiency. Magazine The Journal of Clinical Endocrinology & Metabolism, Volume 95, Issue 8, 1 August 2010, Page E2.

Part IV. Sexual and reproductive disorders

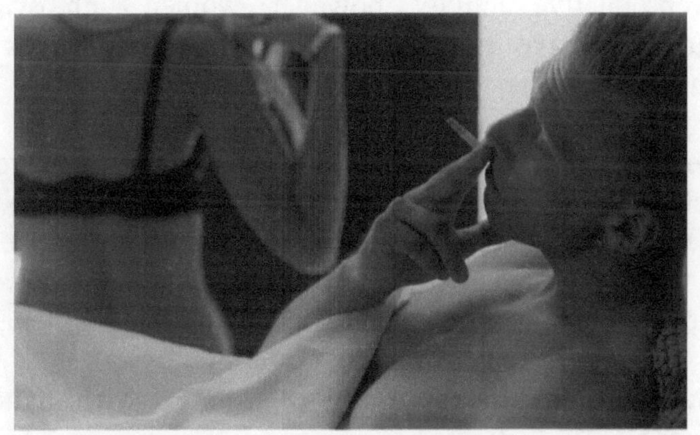

Chapter 22. Primary Ovarian Insufficiency

Primary ovarian insufficiency, also known as premature ovarian failure, is a loss of normal ovarian function before a woman reaches 40 years of age.

This implies that they do not produce normal amounts of estrogen, that ovules are not released every month and that menstruation disappears, therefore pregnancy is impossible.

In general, premature ovarian failure is confused with premature menopause, but in reality they are two different disorders. Premature menopause is the complete cessation of reproductive activity, however, women with ovarian failure may have irregular menstrual periods for years and with treatment they can conceive a child.

As early ovarian failure induces a reduction in the estrogen levels of the affected woman, it is possible that she experiences some complications associated with the lack of this hormone, such as osteoporosis, for example, but proper treatment helps you stay healthy and avoid this problem.

What happens in the body of women with ovarian failure?

Normally in women the pituitary gland releases some hormones during the menstrual cycle that help mature the ovules contained in the ovarian follicles, that happens every month and is repeated until reaching menopause.

When the follicles mature, they open and release an egg that travels to the fallopian tube and awaits a sperm that fertilizes it, but when premature ovarian failure occurs the ovaries do not perform this function and the ovules do not occur so they do not occur performs a menstrual cycle and cannot get pregnant.

What causes premature ovarian failure?

In most cases, the cause of ovarian insufficiency in a patient is unknown, but scientists believe that certain genetic disorders such as Fragile X chromosome syndrome and Turner syndrome increase the chances of ovarian failure.

Exposure to certain toxins, endocrine disruptors, chemotherapy and radiotherapy can damage the genetic material of the cells causing the appearance of ovarian insufficiency, as well as an autoimmune response, in which antibodies attack the ovarian tissue and damage the follicles that contain the ovules. , but in this case the cause of the inverse response of the immune system is also unknown, that is, it is idiopathic.

It is possible that a woman's ovaries manifest a spontaneous failure before reaching forty years of age and have no chromosomal defects, autoimmune diseases, or have been exposed to toxins, in this case your specialist doctor must perform the necessary examinations to find the cause.

According to a study (39) carried out at the Virgen de Valme University Hospital in Seville, smokers have seen an advance of 1-3 years in the onset of natural menopause, but this data lacks weight to justify an insufficiency premature ovarian

Nor has it been shown through research that drinking coffee and alcohol, either excessively or moderately, can increase the chances of this disorder in women.

Bibliography.

(15) López E, Flores A, Romeu S (2010) Study of primary ovarian insufficiency and occult ovarian insufficiency. Available en: https://www.sefertilidad.net/docs/biblioteca/guiasPracticaClinicas/guia 9.pdf

Chapter 23. Menopause

Menopause refer to the changes that an adult woman experiences when she reaches the end of her reproductive capacity. Although it is a normal process, during this stage you can experience various physical and emotional discomforts that are mainly subject to the hormonal changes involved.

The word menopause refers to the specific date on which the woman had her last menstruation and in medical terms it occurs because the ovaries stop producing progesterone and estrogen. Instead, the word climacteric refers to changes that occur in the female body before, during and after menopause.

To determine menopause, twelve consecutive months without menstruation are required, that is, it can only be determined retrospectively and marks the end of fertility. It usually occurs when they are over 50 years of age, but it can also occur after age 42 at an early onset.

As menopause leads to a decrease in hormonal production and the body has several estrogen receptors, in some women certain health problems, such as osteoporosis or the general deterioration of different organs, can be generated.

The decrease in sexual desire, the sensation of suffocation, sleep problems, dry skin and mucous membranes, difficulty concentrating and irritability are symptoms of this period and can be worsened or relieved thanks to habits, environment and stress.

To date it has not been scientifically proven that alcohol can worsen the symptoms of menopause or trigger complications, however, a moderate intake is always recommended, however, tobacco and coffee can influence negatively.

Smokers can advance menopause

Smoking regularly advances the arrival of menopause, that is, shortens the normal reproductive cycle of any woman. This was demonstrated in a study conducted at the Eusebio Hernández Gyneco-Obstetric University Hospital in Cuba (40).

The researchers gathered a group of women between 40 and 59 years old and separated them into perimenopausal and postmenopausal. Each participant's age, age of onset of menopause was obtained, taking into account that this occurred after 12 consecutive months of amenorrhea, marital status, smoking and working condition.

Towards the end of the investigation it was discovered that the menopause age of the women studied was 49.8 years and that it occurred earlier in smokers, at 48.2 years and in those who had no stable partner, which was at 48.3 years.

The interesting thing about this research is that it analyzed other factors besides the cigarette, since the group in charge considered that a single factor cannot be responsible in the alteration of a natural process.

Coffee increases the sensation of suffocation

One of the most annoying and representative symptoms of menopause seems to be exacerbated by caffeine according to a study published in Menopause (41). The research covered more than 1,800 menopausal women between 2005 and 2011, regular consumers and not coffee.

The results reveal that the regulation of the body of the diameter of the blood vessels is altered by caffeine when the woman goes through menopause, and that is why annoying vasomotor symptoms appear, that is, the sudden and temporary appearance of body heat, redness and sweating This generally applies to all caffeinated beverages, such as tea, soda and chocolate.

The recommendations of those in charge of the investigation were to avoid as much as possible the consumption of this type of drinks, maintain a healthy weight, remain active and adopt meditation techniques for the management of emotions. They recognize that it is a stage with many changes and they hope with this information to mitigate the discomforts that women may feel when crossing it.

Bibliografphy.

(16) Braulio Hernández, Miguel L (2007) Age of menopause and its relationship with smoking, marital status and employment. Cuban Journal Obstetrics and Gynecology 2007; 33

(17) Faubion S, Sood R, Jacqueline M, Shuster L (2015) Caffeine and menopausal symptoms what is the association? Menopause Magazine, February 2015 - Volume 22 - Issue 2 - p 155–158

Chapter 24. Female sexual dysfunction

Female sexual dysfunction is a disorder, not a disease, in which there is a pronounced change in a woman's usual sexual behavior. Usually, sexual thoughts and fantasies diminish or disappear, relationships escape and the ability to enjoy intercourse is lost.

When talking about sexual dysfunction in women, we talk about difficulties in four different areas: desire, excitement, orgasm and pain associated with intercourse, also known as dyspareunia.

Disorders of this type can appear at any time in life and can both disappear and become chronic, for example, after a complicated birth, during a very stressful situation or a strong illness, it is likely that the woman will take a Time to be physically active again.

What causes female sexual dysfunction?

It is difficult to establish the causes of the dysfunction since it occurs in very specific areas that often come together in the same patient, however, we will try to understand these factors separately and in a very general way.

• **Loss of desire**: Changes in contraceptive methods, stress, obesity, traumatic sexual episodes, chronic diseases, depression and surgical interventions usually induce the loss of sexual desire in women.

• **Difficulty in arousal:** A physical problem can interfere with blood flow or nerve endings in the genital area as it interferes with messages sent from the genitals to the brain. Similarly, certain coronary diseases and diabetes decrease arousal and prevent the structure of the vagina from being conditioned for penetration.

• Pain associated with intercourse: It may be due to inflammatory diseases of the pelvis, gynecological surgery, tumors, uterine cysts, endometriosis, urinary tract infections, lack of lubrication or any sexually transmitted infection.

• Hormonal problems: Fluctuations in the level of estrogen can cause changes in the genital tissues making them thinner and sensitive to pain, it can also reduce blood circulation to the pelvic region, cause vaginal dryness and make it take more time to reach the excitement and orgasm.

Tobacco adds another factor to the list

According to a statement made at the VII National Meeting of Women's Health and Medicine held in Spain (42), smoking increases the risk of vaginal dryness and genital atrophy, accelerates menopause and decreases estrogen levels. All this significantly accelerates and aggravates hypoactive sexual desire disorder and sexual dysfunction.

In this paper, experts also point out that in 33% of women between 18 and 59 years of age who suffer a decrease in sexual desire, the origin of the problem is mainly psychological, hormonal or a combination of these factors, in other words it is very complex, but smoking only adds one more piece to this apparent puzzle.

What role does alcohol have?

The influence of alcohol on female sexual dysfunction is a bit more complex and science failed to establish a unique theory.

On the one hand, researchers from the University of Salamanca (43) discovered that in alcoholics there are few problems related to sexual dysfunction, in fact, in them sexual functioning in general was acceptable and better in the men studied.

45% of the participants had weekly relationships, 69% experienced sexual desire during the week, 81% of the men had no trouble reaching and maintaining an erection and only 10% suffered premature ejaculation. In the female group only 10% indicated suffering from vaginismus and 5% dyspareunia.

Popular beliefs suggest that alcohol consumption helps us in the process of disinhibition and interacting more openly and this is somehow true, so it may be helpful to drink alcohol, but it can also have the opposite effect depending on explains Dr. Patricia Jordá, a psychologist specializing in Sexual and Couple Therapy.

Alcohol intake may decrease vaginal lubrication, due to the lack of irrigation in the area due to slow circulation and dehydration of the alcohol itself. Similarly, it is likely that orgasm will be delayed or that when it occurs, it will feel less intense due to the sedative effect of alcohol.

Thus, although the intake of alcohol prior to a sexual relationship affects the quality of the act, at the moment it seems that it does not have long-term effects, however, studies are still being carried out that try to solve this disorder that every time It makes more frequent.

Bibliography.

(16) 20 Minutes (2007) Smoking can reduce sexual desire in women and produce vaginal dryness.

Available   en:
https://www.20minutos.es/noticia/206991/0/fumar/
deseo/sexual/

(17) José Ávila, Ana Pérez, Juan Olazábal, Jesús
Fidalgo (2004) Sexual dysfunctions in alcoholism.
Available in: http://www.socidrogalcohol.org

(18) The world (2016) Sex and alcohol, allies or
enemies?   Available   in:
https://www.elmundo.es/promociones/native/2016/
12/17b/

Chapter 25. Endometriosis

Endometriosis is an unpredictable disorder that occurs when cells of the endometrial tissue leave the uterus and develop on the peritoneum, broad ligaments, ovaries, the bottom of the sac, intestine, vagina, cervix, and bladder, In some patients I can even find on the skin and lungs.

The foci where the endometrial tissue lodges respond to the hormones that control the menstrual cycle, therefore, they are sensitive to inflammation and bleed every month but have no possibility of draining the fluid, which accumulates generating scars that deform the surface of the organs and adhere to each other.

In addition to pain, an affected woman may experience dysmenorrhea, dyspareunia, infertility, dysuria and pain during defecation, everything will depend on the location of the ectopic tissue and its development.

Endometriosis occurs in 6-10% of women in general and in 25-50% of women with fertility problems. The average age at which it is diagnosed is around 27 although there is also the possibility that it manifests earlier.

Why does a woman develop endometriosis?

The exact causes of endometriosis are unknown but it is suspected that it is because when a woman has the period a retrograde flow develops whereby the cells return to the pelvis through the fallopian tubes. It is also believed to be due to a failure in the immune system.

In some cases, the woman suffering from endometriosis has a direct relative who also suffers from the disorder, which indicates that there is a genetic condition involved, but has not yet been confirmed through studies.

Women who had early menarche and very long menstrual periods have a higher risk of endometriosis, as do those with closed hymen.

The theory of celomic metaplasia is generally accepted, which explains that by means of a cytological transformation ovarian germ cells and peritoneal cells become endometrial tissue, causing endometriosic lesions.

Alcohol increases the risk significantly

A meta-analysis carried out in the United States and published in the American Journal of Obstetrics and Gynecology (45), showed that there is a risk associated with regular alcohol consumption and the development of endometriosis.

Specifically, according to the findings of the group of researchers, women who were considered frequent drinkers are more prone to the disorder compared to women who did not consume any alcohol.

In addition to this, it was discovered that females with more beverage intake are also more prone to immune and cardiovascular diseases. Thus, a patient with relatives who have suffered endometriosis should refrain from excessive alcohol consumption as it could be a trigger for the condition.

Smoking does not significantly influence

In an article in the journal Fertility and Sterility (46) a group of scientists and doctors made known their findings related to the disease, clarifying that smoking does not increase or reduce the risk of a woman developing endometriosis.

The study used 978 women under 42, 411 of them had the disorder and tissue samples were taken to determine what stage they were in. 45% of the participants of this were smokers or ex-smokers as well as 36% of the 567 women without the disease.

Women without births had the highest rate of endometriosis compared to those who were mothers. It was also shown that thinner women had more risks, but no evidence was found that smoking increased the incidence.

In coffee it affects estrogen and increases the chances

The medical journal American Journal of Clinical Nutrition (47) made a publication in which we can find a relationship between endometriosis and caffeine consumption and that the drink does not directly affect the abnormal development of endometrial tissue, but it can modify hormonal levels and facilitate its appearance.

It seems that caffeine increases estrogen levels in the body and specifically drinking more than two cups of coffee daily can increase the levels of this hormone and increase the chances of the disorder.

One of the researchers in charge of the study explains that variations in estrogen levels are associated with disorders of this type, osteoporosis and endometrial, breast and ovarian cancers, so caffeine consumption should be taken into account in any patient with problems of this type.

Bibliography.

(19) Parazzini F, Cipriani S, Bravi F, Pelucchi C, Chiaffarino F, Ricci E, Viganò P (2013) A metaanalysis on alcohol consumption and risk of endometriosis. Am J Obstet Gynecol. 2013 Aug;209(2):106.e1-10. doi: 10.1016/j.ajog.2013.05.039. Epub 2013 May 23.

(20) Charles C, Carlos S, Dominique Z, Marie-Christine L, Charlotte N, Gérard B, François G, Bruno B (2010) Smoking habits of 411 women with histologically proven endometriosis and 567 unaffected women. Revista Fertility and Sterility olume 94, Issue 6, Pages 2353–2355

(21) Karen C, Enrique F, Sunni L, Anna Z, Cuilin Z, Aijun Y, Joseph B, Ahmad O, Christina A, Jean W (2012) Caffeinated beverage intake and reproductive hormones among premenopausal women in the BioCycle Study. Revista The American Journal of Clinical Nutrition, Volume 95, Issue 2, February 2012, Pages 488–497

Chapter 26. Recurring Abortions

An abortion is the loss of a pregnancy before it reaches twenty-two weeks of gestation or before the fetus reaches 500g of weight. In this situation the fetus dies spontaneously and the mother must receive medical assistance to avoid complications.

On the other hand, a woman is considered to experience recurrent abortions when she loses three or more pregnancies consecutively and spontaneously, as long as they are not ectopic or molar pregnancies, in which the very complex condition of pregnancy induces the expulsion of the fetus in training.

It is estimated that 30% of all pregnancies generally end in a spontaneous abortion, but 20% of them occur before they can be detected by ultrasound. Approximately 5% of women suffer from continuous abortions and in 60% of cases the causes are unknown.

Why do recurrent abortions occur?

The exact causes of recurrent abortions have not been determined, but it is known that in 50% of cases the spontaneous interruption of pregnancy is due to embryonic aneuploidies, that is, a change in the number of chromosomes, which gives Place to genetic diseases.

Age seems to be related to spontaneous abortions and genetic problems because in patients over 40 years of age the probability of embryonic aneuploidy exceeds 80%.
It is believed that women affected with chronic endometriosis are more susceptible to recurrent abortions due to the alteration experienced by endometrial cells, as are patients with uterine fibroids. There is evidence that

myomas distort the endometrial cavity and with this generates a decrease in embryonic implantation.

Recurrent abortions may also be due to infectious, endocrine factors, thyroid abnormalities and diseases such as diabetes mellitus, but the mechanisms by which these conditions prevent a term pregnancy are still unknown.

Tobacco, caffeine and alcohol are linked to abortions in a proportional way, that is, the more you consume the greater the chances, but the evidence is still not enough to be considered a fact.

Coffee and abortion possibilities

In a study published in the British Medical Journal (48), 18,478 Danish women between 1989 and 1996 were analyzed in order to determine their coffee intake. The conclusions reached by the researchers were that pregnant women who consume high doses of this substance recorded twice the risk of having an abortion compared to other women who did not drink coffee.

Each study participant had to fill out two questionnaires specifying their consumption of tobacco, alcohol and caffeinated products, such as tea, chocolate and soda. According to the data obtained, women who ingested little coffee but frequently drank tea and similar products did not have a high risk of losing pregnancy.

In this study, women who drank between four and seven cups of coffee daily recorded an increased risk of abortion by 80%, while those who drank more than eight cups increased the probability by 300%.

The researchers point out that the majority of women with high caffeine consumption were also smokers and drank high doses of alcohol and suspect that the combination of these three factors is a cause with more weight than each element separately.

Smoking and pregnancies that are not carried out

A study conducted in Japan and published by the journal Human Reproduction (49) attempted to show that smoking during pregnancy increases the risk of a miscarriage.

For the analysis, the information of more than 1,300 Japanese women who had had a pregnancy was used and the authors discovered that those women who smoked in large quantities at the beginning of pregnancy were twice as likely to have an abortion during the first trimester than those who did not. smokers

More specifically, women who had smoked at least 20 cigarettes a day during pregnancy were twice as likely as non-smokers to have an abortion, but studies that complement this information are still needed.

Bibliography.

(22) Duro M, Causín S, Campillos P, Vallés U (2001) Caffeine consumption and risk of spontaneous abortion in the first trimester. Medifam vol.11 no.8 Aug./Sep. 2001

(23) Sachiko B (2012) Changes in snuff and smoking habits in Swedish pregnant women and risk for small for gestational age births. BJOG An International Journal of Obstetrics & Gynaecology, November 2012.

Chapter 27. Polycystic Ovarian Syndrome

Polycystic ovary syndrome is a hormonal disorder that occurs when a woman of reproductive age has very high levels of male hormones or androgens.

A high level of androgens in women depresses estrogen and progesterone, which are two female hormones that help the ovaries release eggs ready for fertilization.

This hormonal imbalance in the patient generates accumulations of fluid in the follicles of the ovaries, which results in cysts and the interruption of the menstrual cycle, since mature ovules cannot be released properly. It is also likely to be sterile and your skin will be affected by acne or increased hair. Usually this disorder is detected between the ages of 20 and 30, but it can also affect girls and adolescents with abnormal development, showing symptoms some time after menarche.

Why this problem?

Medicine and science do not yet know the exact cause of polycystic ovary syndrome. These factors are generally considered as risks:

Genetics: Women with polycystic ovaries usually have a mother or sister with similar symptoms.

Little inflammation: According to the Mayo Clinic (50), during an infection the white blood cells generate a certain substance, this is known as "little inflammation". Some women with polycystic ovaries have a low inflammation process that stimulates androgen production and can cause heart problems.

Excess insulin: When cells become resistant to the action of insulin, blood sugar levels rise and the body could produce more insulin.

The excess of this hormone increases the production of androgen, which causes difficulties in the ovulation process.

There is currently no evidence that alcohol, tobacco and coffee are linked to polycystic ovary syndrome. When a woman is diagnosed, she is asked to consume these substances in moderation but it is a general health recommendation.

Bibliography.

(24) Mayo Clinic (2017) Polycystic ovary syndrome. Available in: https://www.mayoclinic.org/es-es/diseases-conditions/pcos/symptoms-causes/syc-20353439

Chapter 28. Female infertility

In terms of medicine, infertility is the inability of a sexually active partner, who is not using contraceptives, to achieve a pregnancy after trying for more than a year. This applies to both male and female gender because 35% of the time infertility comes from problems in women and 35% of men.

A pregnancy, however common it may seem, involves a series of biological mechanisms, for example, in the ovaries of the woman a healthy ovum must be produced, just as in the seminiferous tubes of the man, healthy sperm must be produced.

The healthy egg must be collected by one of the fallopian tubes and await a fertilizing sperm, once this happens both move to the uterus and begins the process of cell division that will give rise to the fetus. It is enough that one of these or other steps not mentioned is interrupted or affected in some way to stop a pregnancy.

What can cause female infertility?

There are many reasons why a woman is not fertile but summarizing could be due to disorders of the menstrual cycle, abnormalities of the fallopian tubes or uterus, endometriosis, cervical mucus problems, stress, sexuality disorders, chronic diseases, age and weight.

In 12% of cases, primary infertility is due to problems with women's weight. Thus, extreme loss of body weight and certain disorders such as anorexia nervosa decrease the chances of conceiving a child.

Excessive sports activity on the other hand, also alters the hormonal balance and reduces fertility, as well as the overweight that causes the sending of abnormal hormonal signals that affects ovulation and is associated with problems such as polycystic ovary syndrome.

The consumption of certain substances also affects the delicate biological balance that must exist for the female body to achieve a conception, let's see how.

Tobacco ages the reproductive system

Women who smoke have more problems getting pregnant than non-smoking women, and this is directly proportional to the amount of tobacco consumed daily, even passively.

Spain is a country where assisted reproduction has become very important, in fact, 3% of children born in this country are the product of medical interventions to reach conception. Victoria Verdú (51), a renowned doctor and coordinator of the assisted reproduction clinic Ginefiv, clearly explains the relationship between cigarette toxicity and infertility.

The substances present in tobacco deteriorate the female reproductive system to the point that it seems to be ten years older because it has a worse ovocitary and embryonic quality.

Women are born with a specific number of ovules that will ripen and be released during their fertile life, this is known as ovarian reserve, nicotine, cyanide and carbon monoxide from cigarettes accelerate the loss of immature ovules, this is why Smoking anticipates the arrival of menopause.

Similarly, these substances damage the genetic material, increase the risk of miscarriage, premature births, ectopic pregnancies and reduce the success rates of assisted reproduction treatment such as artificial insemination and in vitro fertilization.

Alcohol also decreases ovarian reserve

Another great specialist in assisted reproduction from the Bernabeu Institute (52) explains that alcohol decreases the ovarian reserve when its intake is exceeded, more specifically, the daily consumption of 2-3 alcoholic beverages multiplies the risk of infertility by 1.6.

Alcohol causes ovulation problems because it alters the hormonal regulation of the normal ovarian cycle, it also increases the abortion rate, low birth weight and fetal death.

The effects of alcohol have repercussions in both genders but it seems that women are more susceptible to having a faster gastrointestinal absorption and a slower metabolization through the enzyme alcohol dehydrogenase.

Caffeine recovers the movement in the fallopian tubes

Finally there is coffee, whose effect on fertility was unknown until recently when a brilliant publication was made in the British Journal of Pharmacology (53).

As we saw at the beginning of the chapter, to achieve a pregnancy, the ovules must travel from the ovaries to the uterus. This path involves cilia or microscopic villi present in the lining of the oviducts and muscular contractions in the inner walls of the tubes.

These contractions are carried out with the help of specialized cells, called pacemaker cells and caffeine stops this function so that the eggs enter a state similar to rest and this already represents

Bibliography.

(24) Victoria Verdú (2013) Smoking halves the chances of pregnancy. Available:https://www.efesalud.com/fumar-reduce-a-la-mitad-las-posibilidades-de-gestacion/

(25) Lydia Luque (2018) The effects of alcohol on fertility. Available in:https://www.institutobernabeu.com/foro/los-efectos-del-alcohol-en-la-fertilidad/

(26) RE Dixon, SJ Hwang, FC Britton, KM Sanders, SM Ward (2011) Inhibitory effect of caffeine on pacemaker activity in the oviduct is mediated by cAMP-regulated conductances. Revista British Journal of Pharmacol. 2011 Jun; 163(4): 745–754.

Chapter 29. Male Infertility

Male infertility is the inability of a man to get a woman pregnant after having had sex for a year without using any kind of protection. As we saw, in 35% of cases of infertile couples, problems revolve around man.

As with female fertility, there are many conditions that affect male gametes, for example, a low sperm production, that they have very low quality or quantity in the ejaculate and that they have abnormal behavior, but this can only Be diagnosed by a fertility medical exam.

A lower than normal sperm count is around 15 million sperm per milliliter of semen or a total sperm count approaches 39 million by ejaculation.

Why is a man sterile?

Chronic health problems, injuries to the testicles or scrotum and having a retained testicle can cause male infertility, as well as erectile dysfunction and difficulty ejaculating.

Receiving a lot of heat in the testicles by wearing tight clothes or, on the contrary, being exposed to too cold for a long time, affects the quality of the semen because the spermatogenesis occurs in a fairly reduced temperature range and once it leaves it The process is not carried out correctly.

Most men ignore the fact that they are infertile, unless they are willing to conceive a child, since the symptoms are sometimes not evident and when they do they are associated with other diseases.

Thus, an infertile man may have pain, swelling and a lump in the testicles, recurrent respiratory infections, gynecomastia and decreased facial and body hair and these problems may or may not be associated with infertility.

Exposure to certain substances that act as endocrine disruptors, alter the hormonal balance and are largely responsible for fertility problems and as we will see below, the consumption of coffee, alcohol and tobacco also have a certain negative effect.

Coffee can damage sperm structure

In a recent study conducted at Massachusetts General Hospital (54), it was shown that caffeine could damage sperm at the molecular level, which would cause problems in the quality of a man's sperm.

The investigators in charge evaluated samples from a group of 105 men with an average of 37 years of age destined for an assisted fertility treatment, more specifically, their partner received in vitro fertilization.

The results showed that volunteers who drank two or more daily cups of strong coffee per day had only 1 in 5 chances of success in treatment, but men who drank less than one cup daily increased the chance to 52%.

According to Anatte Karmon, one of the researchers, the high consumption of caffeine in men seems to reduce the chances of the couple getting a clinical pregnancy and therefore a mandatory measure for assisted fertility is adequate nutrition.

Smoking mothers can make their children sterile

It has long been proven that smoking reduces men's fertility, causes impotence and damages sperm, but what was ignored is that the children of smoking mothers could also have trouble conceiving a child in adulthood.

In a study conducted at the University of Copenhagen (55) the embryos of women who had legally aborted were analyzed and it was found that in the fetuses of smoking mothers there were 55% less germ cells, which form the semen and the ovules, and 37% less somatic cells, from which other parts of the body are formed.

It was also discovered that the reduction in the amount of both types of cells is directly related to the number of cigarettes that are smoked daily and that this effect is more intense in males than in females.

In conclusion, children born to women smokers may have fertility problems by having a smaller number of germ cells and it is not known if they will eventually recover the full functionality of the testicles.

Alcohol makes sperm quality worse

Research published in the British Medical Journal shows that young people who consume alcohol regularly have a worse seminal quality as they get older.

To prove it, the scientists used the data of 1,221 men between the ages of 18 and 28, who conducted a questionnaire about their alcohol consumption habits, specifying how often they consumed it and the amount of drinks. After solving these questions, his semen was analyzed along with his reproductive hormonal capacity.

The results indicate that the participants consumed an average of 11 drinks per week, 64% of them had got drunk the previous month and 59% had got drunk more than twice.

In these men testosterone levels had increased, while the sex hormone binding globulin (SHBG), which activates sex hormones, had been significantly reduced, in addition, in the total sperm count and the proportion thereof, the men who obtained worse results were those who abused the drink.

Bibliography.

(27) Tina Kold Jensen, Mads Gottschau, Jens Otto Broby Madsen, Anne-Maria Andersson, Tina Harmer Lassen, Niels E Skakkebæk, Shanna H Swan, Lærke Priskorn, Anders Juul, Niels Jørgensen (2014) Regular alcohol consumption associated with reduced semen quality and changes in reproductive hormones; a cross-sectional study among 1221 young Danishmen. British Medical Journal magazine. Available at: https://bmjopen.bmj.com/content/4/9/e005462

(28) L.S. Mamsen, Lutterodt, E.W. Andersen, S.O. Skouby, K.P. Sørensen, C. Yding Andersen, A.G. Byskov (2010) Cigarette smoking during early pregnancy reduces the number of embryonic germ and somatic cells Human Reproduction, Volume 25, Issue 11, November 2010, Pages 2755–2761

(29) National post (2014) Coffee consumption linked to male infertility, U.S. study suggests. Available at: https://nationalpost.com/health/coffee-consumption-linked-to-male-infertility-u-s-study-suggests

Chapter 30. Gynecomastia

Gynecomastia is the term used to refer to the excessive development of the breast or breast in men. This physical abnormality occurs in response to too much estrogen, which is a predominantly female hormone and too little testosterone, which is in greater numbers in the male gender.

When gynecomastia is suffered, the glandular tissue of the breast swells and forms a breast button, this is known as breast hypertrophy. According to the Spanish Society of Reconstructive and Aesthetic Plastic Surgery (SECPRE) between 40 and 60% of men of all ages, from babies to older adults (57)

What causes gynecomastia?

There are several factors that can develop this condition, for example, the use of certain medications, such as prednisone, cimetidine and phenytoin. Also the use of chemotherapy drugs and antidepressants.

Exposure to certain substances that alter the endocrine system and the use of psychotropic substances can increase breast development in a man, as well as hormonal mismatches of his age.

Teenagers may experience gynecomastia due to the changes their body experiences, but in this case it disappears on its own in a period of six to twenty four months.

In newborn babies, a breast button may occur because of their mother's estrogen levels and in this case it will also disappear naturally after half a year.

In adult men, gynecomastia is associated with serious conditions, such as liver or lung cancer, cirrhosis of the liver, an overactive thyroid and hormonal problems.

Does it influence what is consumed?

Currently there is not enough evidence to show that coffee, smoking and alcohol can generate gynecomastia, however, it is considered that excess drinks could be related.

Alcohol consumption causes testosterone levels in men to decrease and as an natural response of the body there is an increase in estrogen, decrease in sexual desire and impotence.

It is believed that prolonged contamination of the body with alcohol creates greater opportunities for estrogen to accumulate and gynecomastia develop, but this has not been demonstrated through scientific studies.

Bibliography.

(30) Health (2019) Gynecomastia, abnormal growth of breasts in a male, affects between 40 and 60% of men. Available in:http://isanidad.com/146322/la-ginecomastia-es-el-crecimiento-anormal-de-las-mamas-en-un-varon-afecta-a-entre-un-40-y-60-de-hombres/

Chapter 31. Erectile Dysfunction

Erectile dysfunction, also known as impotence, is the persistent inability to get an erection or maintain it with the firmness necessary to have a sexual relationship. It is a problem that affects more than 50% of men over the age of 40, but it can also occur in young people around twenty.

In general, a man with impotence may have an erection on certain occasions, but not every time he wishes to have sex, he may also have an erection, but not for the time necessary to successfully conclude a sexual relationship, others may not have an erection in no time.

Having erection problems occasionally is not synonymous with suffering from erectile dysfunction, only when it ceases to be a punctual event and is repeated for a minimum period of three months is that it should be considered a health problem because sometimes it is a problem related to others serious pathologies

What causes erectile dysfunction?

An erection is the response to male sexual arousal, which is a complex process in which the brain, emotions, hormones, nerves, muscles and blood vessels are involved, when one of these factors presents a problem, the erectile dysfunction.

It can also be the result of a problem of chronic stress, anxiety, the consumption of certain medications or some physical illness that makes the sexual response slower, for example, a problem in the circulatory, vascular or endocrine system.

Obesity, type 2 diabetes, atherosclerosis, high blood pressure, Peyronie's disease NIH external link, a lesion in the penis, spinal cord, prostate, bladder or pelvis can also cause this problem. Some men have difficulty maintaining an erection as they get older, however, old age is not a cause of erectile dysfunction.

Coffee can improve this condition

A study carried out by the Center for Health Sciences at the University of Texas at Houston (58), has found that coffee and, in general, caffeine-containing drinks can improve impotence problems.

The investigation reviewed information from the National Health and Nutrition Examination Survey program, in which 3,724 men over 20 years of age and with impotence problems participated. Of these men, 40.9% were overweight, 30.7% obese, 51% high blood pressure and 12.4% diabetes.

The results of the analysis revealed that those who consumed 2 or 3 cups of coffee a day were 42% less likely to have erectile dysfunction or impotence, regardless of their health condition, compared to those who did not drink any caffeine or less than one Cup. This effect cannot be seen in the diabetics of the study.

The researchers do not know what is the exact mechanism of action of caffeine on dysfunction but they suspect that they cause relaxation of the arteries of the penis and the cavernous smooth muscle, thereby increasing blood flow and allowing erection.

Tobacco and alcohol are not friends of erections

Boston Medical Group is a worldwide alliance of medical clinics specializing in the treatment of male sexual dysfunctions and have carried out an investigation with 447 men suffering from erectile dysfunction, their ages were between 18 and 35 years.

In their investigation they discovered that in 62.5% of the cases the main cause was the excessive consumption of alcohol, even if they were not alcoholic patients. They explain the following: The drink slows, distorts and slows the perception and response of our senses as reflexes, vision, hearing and sexual response, as it depresses the functioning of the central nervous system. This is a direct consequence of alcohol consumption, which is why it occurs both in punctual intake and in those who maintain the habit, but in alcoholics these disorders become chronic and sometimes irreversible.

This study also revealed that tobacco is responsible for erectile dysfunction by 16.5% and this is due to the progressive obstruction it causes in veins and arteries, while some drugs such as cocaine, a central nervous system stimulant, they act as vasoconstrictor, reducing blood flow in veins and arteries

Bibliografía.

(31) López DS, Liu L, Rimm EB, Tsilidis KK, de Oliveira Otto M, Wang R, Canfield S, GiovannucciE (2018) CoffeeIntake and Incidence of ErectileDysfunction. Revista Am J Epidemiol. 2018 May 1;187(5):951-959. doi: 10.1093/aje/kwx304.

(32) Boston Medical Group (2012) Disfunción eréctil en hombres. Disponible en:

https://www.bostonmedicalgroup.es/estudios-disfuncion-erectil/alcohol-y-disfuncion-erectil-jovenes

Chapter 32. Andropause

Andropause is the gradual decrease in testosterone production. It usually manifests itself in men once they reach forty years of age and it is a natural and slow progression process in which the ability to procreate is lost, that is, to get a woman pregnant.

This condition is associated with aging and does not manifest itself in all men in the same way, as some may conceive a child even at age 70, others may not change and as it is not a process so marked and defined science and The medicine has not been studied as carefully as menopause, and the symptoms are not as clear.

A man who goes through menopause experiences sleep disturbances, genital hair loss, depression, irritability, lack of concentration, constant fatigue, headache, low ejaculation power, decreased libido, dry scalp and skin and night sweats .

All these symptoms can be associated with other health conditions or misunderstood with stress. Only a hormonal test would show that it is a decrease in the hormone testosterone and this after fifty years is lost between 1% - 2% every year (60).

Can andropause be accelerated or delayed?

Andropause is a natural process, since all living organisms must experience the cessation of their reproductive functions as part of the normal cycle of life, however, not all men manifest themselves equally.

In some men the symptoms of andropause are accentuated and they interrupt the performance of their activities, their mood and vitality so artificial treatment is necessary to increase their hormonal level, but this is done based on the baseline levels that the patient would be for his age.

Some factors can negatively affect the process and make the symptoms more annoying, then some of them:

• Anxiety, stress and depression.
• Bad habits and an unhealthy lifestyle.
•Obesity and overweight
• Chronic diseases such as diabetes and hypertension
• Problems in the function of the hypothalamus

There is no evidence that excessive consumption of coffee, alcohol and tobacco have a negative effect on men with andropause, however, general medical recommendations are always aimed at moderation, especially when it comes to these substances that could cause other diseases.

Bibliography.

(33) Marina García (2018) Andropausia, the male menopause. Available in the digital review:https://www.webconsultas.com/tercera-edad/la-salud-del-mayor/en-que-consiste-la-andropausia

Epilogue: Alerts and recommendations

As it was commented at the beginning of the book, it is not easy to establish a single dose of coffee or alcohol, or to affirm to a patient, "you can drink calmly", because in some cases these substances are not responsible for a specific disease, but in others.

When we look around, we may see people whose intake of coffee or alcohol is much higher than that mentioned in the studies cited and seem to be far from suffering the disease, such is the case of older adults who had many children and their fertility was not affected by the excessive intake of coffee.

Science only seeks a solution to the health problems that are becoming more frequent every day in our society and the studies of today are made to people who lived in conditions different from those of many decades ago, so it is not surprising that things that are hard to believe are currently demonstrated.

In the case of cigarettes, we could say that it is the only substance that we should avoid, since it contains so many toxic chemicals that we would hardly get anything beneficial from it, it is also not necessary.

If your desire is to drink coffee and alcohol in moderation, remember to take into account your current health condition, the diseases described in this book and the recommendation of your GP. If you constantly monitor your health, maintain healthy habits, drink in moderation and occasionally will not affect your health with the appearance of any pathology or disorder.

About the Author

Mario Vega Carbó

- Cuban doctor graduated in 1994.
- Specialist in Endocrinology and Family Medicine.
- Master in Longevity and Ultrasonography.
- Professor of Medical Pathophysiology.
- Lover of doing good, family and nature.

Other books of the author

1. An approach to Natural Endocrinology
2. Endocrine Alerts: Saving Lives
3. ABC of the Endocrinologist, for the non-specialist
4. Recipes of your Endocrine
5. Where hormone queen ... short stories
6. Food myths, vision of the Endocrinologist
7. S.O.S Hormonal toxins, naked truths
8. Vitamin D: An omnipresent hormone?
9. Hormones, exercises and fitness body
10. Obesity, Diabetes, Thyroid and S.O.P

Available in 10 languages!

Social Media:

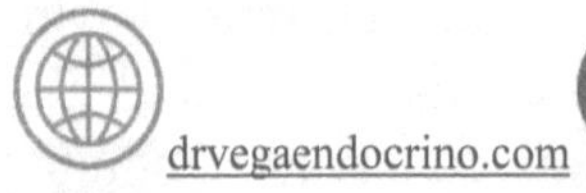 drvegaendocrino.com

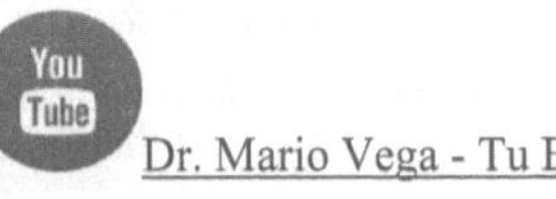 Dr. Mario Vega - Tu Endocrino Online

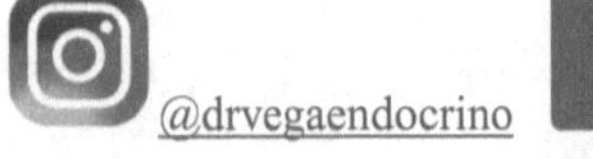 @drvegaendocrino

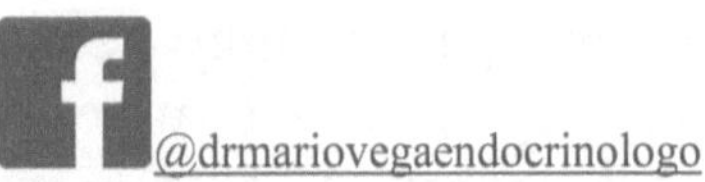 @drmariovegaendocrinologo

Synopsis

"A sporadic drink does not hurt anyone ... a cup of coffee in the morning is what I need to start my day ... the cigar keeps me thin...", some of these ideas may be present in our daily conversations with friends, But the reality is that all these compounds are legal drugs whose effects may be more harmful than beneficial under certain conditions.

To clarify these doubts, Dr. Mario Vega Carbó presents ***"Coffee, tobacco and alcohol: Theirs metabolic and hormonal disorders"***, a book with all the necessary explanations to know what are the real benefits of the world's most popular social drugs.

In this text, we are going to analyze the possible causes and general consequences for health, specifically about the metabolic and hormonal disorders of the habits of consuming coffee, tobacco and alcohol in healthy people, with health risk or with some nutritional, endocrine or reproductive

In just four sections, with more than thirty chapters, truly learn what you consume and what the effects are, know all the secrets of coffee, tobacco and alcohol, in this new book by Dr. Mario Vega Carbó.